THE 20/20 LIFESTYLES METABOLIC CURE

YOUR CLEAR PATH TO REVERSING HIGH CHOLESTEROL, HYPERTENSION, DIABETES AND ENJOYING PERMANENT WEIGHT LOSS

Mark Dedomenico, MD
Barry Wolborsky, PhD

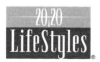

Published by PRO Sports Club, Bellevue and Seattle, Washington.
In association with Better Life Press, Seattle Washington.

proclub.com
2020LifeStyles.com

ISBN: Hardback: 978-0-9909514-0-7

Metadata: 1 Health/fitness. 2 Diet/exercise/nutrition. 3 Metabolic disease, high cholesterol, hypertension, heart disease, diabetes. 4 Weight loss/weight management. 5 Reversing metabolic disease/natural permanent weight loss. 6 Mark Dedomenico, MD, cardiovascular surgeon, researcher, author. 7 Barry Wolborsky, PhD, psychologist, addictions expert, author.

Cover design: Molly Owen
Interior layout design: Molly Owen

This book is dedicated to the staff of the 20/20 LifeStyles program who have lengthened and improved the lives of over 10,000 individuals.

TABLE OF CONTENTS

CHAPTER 4: TAKING CONTROL

CHAPTER 5: THE CHEMISTRY OF OBESITY

CHAPTER 6: THE SELF-SLIMMING MINDSET

CHAPTER 7: REAPING THE REWARDS

CHAPTER 8: NOW, FOR THE NEW LIFESTYLE

CHAPTER 9: LET'S GET INTO ACTION

CHAPTER 10: LEARNING ABOUT YOUR BODY

CHAPTER 11: LEARNING ABOUT YOUR BODY

CHAPTER 12: PUTTING IT ALL TOGETHER

CHAPTER 13: WELCOME TO YOUR FUTURE-MAINTAINING YOUR WEIGHT LOSS AND YOUR NEW HEALTH

CHAPTER 14: THE NUGGETS-LIFE LESSONS THAT LAST

APPENDIX: RESOURCES FOR HEALTH

ACKNOWLEDGEMENTS

The authors wish to thank Andy Miller MS, RD, CD for the enormous effort that she expended organizing the nutritional information and recipes and helping to simplify a complex subject. We also would like to thank Clark Masterson MS, CSCS for his input on exercise and how to keep it safe for beginners.

We are also grateful to Judy Crane and Jen Masterson for keeping us on track and dealing with the mega re-writes that created this book.

Additionally, to our panel of community physicians who carefully read the manuscript and helped us shape this book to the needs of their patients; thank you.

Lastly, we would like acknowledge the staff of the 20/20 LifeStyles Program, the Counseling Center at PRO Sports Club and all the dietitians, counselors, physicians and exercise physiologists at PRO Sports Club who carefully read this book and gave us the feedback we needed to correct errors and include the important details we had omitted. Thank you all!

20/20 LIFESTYLES STAGES GUIDE

The 20/20 LifeStyles nutrition plan is based upon a modified elimination diet. The meal plans follow a multi-staged approach in which food groups are gradually re-introduced as you progress through the program, to teach appropriate portion size and identify any food intolerances or sensitivities. These nutritionally-balanced meal plans are carefully designed by registered dietitians for each individual to help you achieve weight loss and correct metabolic conditions such as high cholesterol, high blood pressure, and type 2 diabetes with effective lifestyle changes.

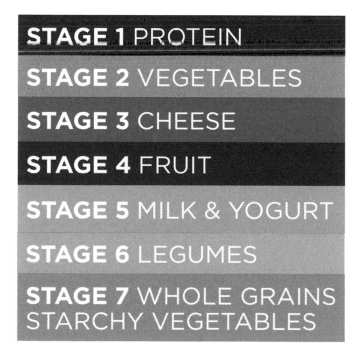

STAGE 1 PROTEIN

STAGE 2 VEGETABLES

STAGE 3 CHEESE

STAGE 4 FRUIT

STAGE 5 MILK & YOGURT

STAGE 6 LEGUMES

STAGE 7 WHOLE GRAINS STARCHY VEGETABLES

INTRODUCTION TO HEALTH

If you want to lose weight and keep it off, then this book is for you. You will learn how to correct your cholesterol and blood pressure levels, reverse your type 2 diabetes and enjoy good health. The sole purpose of this book is to enable the individual who has tried and failed at diets to finally lose weight and maintain the weight loss. This book is not for those who still believe in the "magic" of fad diets. It is for those who are willing to follow instructions and change their life and their lifestyle, so they may enjoy the gifts of a slim, strong, healthy body.

In my practice as a cardiovascular surgeon, I saw the results of metabolic disease. I worked with patients who would have given anything to correct the damage an unhealthy lifestyle had caused. Often I was able to help these extremely ill people; sometimes I was not able to help. I saw this parade of the consequences of unhealthy lifestyle daily, yet I myself weighed 275 pounds at 6 foot 1. Worse yet, I had developed high blood pressure, high cholesterol, and type 2 diabetes.

I rationalized that as a surgeon I worked long hours and had no time for cooking, exercise, or sleep. But the reality is that my lifestyle was just as bad as that of the patients I was operating on every day.

I became very focused on finding a way of correcting the lifestyle that was killing me and my patients. The result was the 20/20 LifeStyles program at the PRO Sports Club in Bellevue, Washington. For 20-plus years, I have worked that program with a team of highly skilled medical doctors, psychologists, dietitians, and exercise physiologists. We have modified, improved, and added to that program and now count more than 10,000 individuals who have successfully changed their lifestyles to achieve normal weight, fitness, and health. I'd like to think our efforts have kept many, many people out of the offices of cardiovascular surgeons. And, by the way, at a very muscular 205 pounds, with normal blood pressure, cholesterol, and blood sugar level, I am one of them.

Our society is being devastated by obesity and the metabolic cascade of diseases caused by obesity. You have been given inadequate information and bad information regarding nutrition and metabolic disease. You see so much conflicting information that you don't know where to turn or what to believe. You see so many websites, books, supplements, TV and magazine ads that you're almost paralyzed by the choices. Many of you are so confused and hopeless that you just give up.

For more than 20 years, we have treated patients with obesity and other metabolic disorders at the 20/20 LifeStyles program at PRO Sports Club in Bellevue, Washington. Our physicians, registered dietitians, exercise physiologists, and lifestyle counselors have successfully treated more than 10,000 individuals just like you. This book is not based on theory or some bright idea. It's based on medical science and our 20-year experience of discovering the most effective treatments to reverse and permanently control obesity and other metabolic disorders.

In order for you to be successful at controlling your weight, a profound change must occur in your perceptions, attitudes, and self-talk. Your feelings about yourself can either enable your success or lead to repeated failures. Hence, much of this book is designed to give you the tools necessary to modify those feelings.

If you are to be in complete control of your health, it is important for you to understand some fairly complex nutritional, medical, and psychological concepts. In this book, we present you with all the information you will need, and we have tried to present it in a simplified way that makes it easy to understand and use.

Chapters 1 through 8 present the medical, scientific, psychological, and nutritional basis for the changes you'll be making. These are critical chapters, because they enable you to make the changes necessary for success on the 20/20 LifeStyles plan. Without the information in these chapters, you will just be following another "diet." And even though it is a well-planned, nutritional diet, without the information in Chapters 1 through 8 you will not be able to achieve long-term success.

Chapters 9 through 12 provide step-by-step instructions for the nutritional, exercise, and lifestyle portions of this plan. As soon as you feel ready to begin your health and weight-loss journey, feel free to skip to Chapter 9 and begin Stage 1 of the plan. At this point it is a good idea for you to look at our meal tracker on the web: www.2020lifestyles.com/get-started/get-started-online/track-it.aspx

But remember, DO NOT stop reading the previous chapters.

Chapter 13 is the maintenance chapter. In this chapter you will learn how to maintain your new body and health for the long term. The chapter explains what you need to do daily and what to do "when the wheels come off" and you find yourself in trouble with your eating.

Chapter 14 is a summary of the gems to take away from this book. These are the most important principles for your new life and happiness.

The appendixes include recipes and resources for those of you who wish to delve more deeply into some of the subjects presented in the previous chapters.

Throughout this book certain guidelines or concepts are repeated. These are the points we think are critical to your success, so if you are reading something for the second or third time, please be sure to take note of it.

This is a "hands-on" book. It is designed as an instruction manual so you can lose weight, maintain that weight loss, and rise to your peak of health and fitness. In order to facilitate that, we have included a number of assignments. For best results, you should complete those assignments at the time you read them. We have found that putting off assignments until later leads to poor results.

Chapters 1-8, 13, and 14 begin with the personal stories of just a few of the 10,000 people who have successfully completed the 20/20 LifeStyles program, which is the basis of this book. You may identify with some of these stories. They can inspire you and give you hope because others just like you have changed their lives and are enjoying long-term health and happiness.

After the stories, in most chapters, you will find concept sections. These twenty-three concepts are your step-by-step roadmap to the self-slimming mindset.

We'll begin with the story of Donna, how she discovered her self-slimming mindset and progressed from deep despair to joy.

CHAPTER 1

LESSONS IN SELF-LOVE AND EMOTIONAL SURVIVAL

MY DESCENT INTO DARKNESS
Donna, age 36

I hated my life. One day was just the same as the next, and there was no change in sight. I was depressed and had been depressed for a long time.

After all, I was permanently single, lonely, unhappy, and fat.

I covered up my misery pretty well. No one really knew how bad it was, although my closest friends knew I wasn't very happy.

My life hadn't turned out as I'd hoped. Dreams of white picket fences and handsome princes were replaced with the realities of a mundane job and comfort food. My feelings of giving up on life became more persistent as the years progressed.

On this particular Friday, I had called in sick because I was too depressed to go to work. As I prepared to spend my weekend alone as usual, I had reached my lowest point.

It was a few minutes before 6:00 p.m.

I was wearing my favorite oversized sweatshirt, one of the few items that still fit me, cradling my third glass of Chardonnay in my right hand as I paced around the house trying to drown the thoughts of the previous evening's disaster.

My best friend, Laura, had set me up on a blind date. Prior to the date, I had gone shopping to find the perfect dress, hoping a new outfit would bring me a spark of luck in the romance department. I hated shopping for clothes. Everything I liked was too snug, hugging my frame too tightly in all the wrong places. Items that did fit were amorphous in shape and more resembled a tent than an outfit. I hated going to the "big girl" department, but after going to many stores, spending many hours and with a bit of luck, I found a black dress that made me feel like I had a figure.

I had spent hours getting ready for this date and was feeling hopeful. When my date arrived, tall and handsome, my heart fluttered with hope and excitement. His body language upon seeing me didn't reflect the same sentiments. After an awkward handshake and shallow small talk over appetizers, I was sure this date would end like all the others, which meant me home alone with Ben and Jerry to dull the blow of another failed evening.

My suspicions were confirmed when my "prince not-so-charming" didn't even finish his dinner before his cell phone rang. Moments later he left, apologizing that he had to go take care of his sick mother. Convenient timing, right?

When you're only 5 feet 3 and 180 pounds, you look and feel fat. To make matters worse, I hadn't gone to the gym in years, so I was seriously out of shape. I had a soft, prematurely aged appearance. Most people thought I must be 45, even though I was only in my mid-30s.

Just two weeks before, I'd seen my primary care doctor for severe headaches. Doctor Mary Roberts spent a lot of time with me, which showed me that she truly cared about my well-being. She told me I had a sinus infection and started me on antibiotics. Then she proceeded to tell me what every other doctor had told me: I needed to lose 50-60 pounds. She was also concerned that my blood pressure was too high. She gave me two choices: go on medication or lose weight. She recommended losing weight, and to appease her, I said I would. She referred me to Dr. Mark Dedomenico, who had a special program for weight loss and metabolic disorders like high blood pressure. She said she would send him my medical records and asked that I call him for an appointment.

Even before I left Dr. Roberts's office I knew I wouldn't make that call. I'd been on every diet known to man, with zero success. There was no hope for me when it came to diets, and I had accepted that. I dismissed the idea of making the phone call and subjecting myself to another failure.

I was at my lowest point. I was sitting on my bed, too miserable to cry and just looking off into space.

There, on my nightstand, I saw an aging framed picture of me with my parents. I looked at their smiling faces, filled with love and joy. I knew my parents loved me, but much of the time that love was shown with food. There were special foods for special occasions, a special meal for my consistently high grades at school, a family dinner out when I won academic awards.

As tears welled up in my eyes, I realized I hadn't felt loved in a long time. My parents were both gone-Dad with a heart attack at 55, Mom with a stroke at 61.

In the photo I saw my 250-pound Dad, my 190-pound Mom, and a chubby little girl that was me. No wonder I was doomed. I had been brilliant at work and at school, but at managing my life and weight I was a complete failure.

My dieting history started when I was a teenager. I noticed my body didn't look like the other girls in my class. They got the boys' attention, and I didn't. When you're a 5-1, 145-pound 15-year-old, you don't fit in.

While school was brutal, P.E. was my personal nightmare. Those tiny athletic shorts only made my excessive size more apparent, and my lack of coordination just worsened my shame.

My parents saw my unhappiness and were willing to send me to any program that could help. I tried every fad diet that came out but never made it a week. I went to a doctor and got shots. Still no help. I tried every national weight-loss program and failed at them all. Every time I failed, my hope dwindled as my self-loathing grew. My long, frustrating, weight-loss journey-to-nowhere had brought me to this moment. I couldn't face another failure. I was hopeless.

My head was hurting again, and I reached into my purse for the Tylenol but couldn't find them. Frustrated and angry, I dumped the purse out on the bed and found the pills. As I reached for them, I saw the note from Dr. Roberts, referring me to Dr. Dedomenico's clinic.

I'm not a very religious person, but I felt that seeing that note at this particular time was some sort of sign.

There must have been some spark of survival instinct left in me, because I picked up the note. When you're at your bottom, you have nothing to lose, so I dialed the number.

Little did I know that because of the hour, Dr. Dedomenico's staff had gone home.

A voice answered, though: "Hello."

I whispered, "Hello, can I speak to Doctor Dedomenico? My name is Donna, and I've been referred to him by Doctor Roberts."

The unfamiliar voice on the other end said, "Hi, Donna, this is Doctor Dedomenico. It's been a couple of weeks since Doctor Roberts referred you to our clinic. You haven't called, and I was concerned."

Knowing this could be my last chance, when I responded to him, I was completely honest. "Doctor, I didn't call because I didn't want to live through another failure. I just couldn't stand that." The sincerity poured out of me. "I've been overweight since I was five. I've been on every diet there is, and it hasn't done any good. I'm a hopeless case."

In a caring, nonjudgmental voice, Dr. Dedomenico said, "Donna, can I ask you something?"

I thought, here we go, here comes the onslaught of questions about my weight, what I eat, etc. But I responded, "I guess so."

To my surprise, he asked, "Do you love yourself?"

I was shocked. I didn't know how to answer.

After a few seconds, Dr. Dedomenico repeated the question. "I hope you don't mind me asking. Do you love yourself?"

During the long pause that followed, my thoughts were reeling, while he said nothing. Finally I said, "Doctor, it's been a very long time since I loved myself. I don't know where or when it went away, but it's gone. For years, I think I have been substituting food for love, and it has never worked. I don't even like myself. Actually, I feel the world would be a better place without me."

Feeling hopeless, I began to cry.

His voice was steady, reassuring. "Donna, you are not alone. Many of the people we work with have felt exactly the same way you feel right now. We have a very caring and loving staff. We care about every single individual we help, and we will love you, until you learn to love yourself. We'll love you no matter what your weight is. We'll love you no matter what your medical condition. We'll love you no matter what shape you are in. And, we'll love you even if you can't be perfect all the time."

His words were so heartfelt and sincere that my hopes rose as he went on. "I'm giving a seminar[1] on Thursday night from six to eight-thirty p.m., and I've saved a seat for you. Will you come?"

I virtually leapt at the opportunity and answered, "Yes, yes I will." And I meant it. If a complete stranger could care that much about me, I needed to care enough about myself to show up. I didn't know it then, but with that one word, "Yes," I had started to change. As I would soon realize, being able to accept myself and then respect myself were the first steps in learning to love myself. For once, the hope I felt had begun to lift my deep depression.

But later as I sat in my car in the parking lot of the health club, my firm conviction began to evaporate. All I could think of were those miserable days in my P.E. class. My mind wanted me to drive away, but my hands wouldn't reach for the key. To make matters worse, I couldn't stop sweating.

I forced myself out of the car, fearful that everyone in the building would look like Jillian Michaels. I entered the lobby on shaky legs, and before I had time to turn back, a smiling woman greeted me and asked if I was there for the 20/20 LifeStyles seminar. I reluctantly answered that I was. As she led me down the hall, I noticed the people around me weren't like Jillian after all; they all looked like normal people.

We finally entered a large lecture hall. Most seats were already filled. Anticipation and nervous energy filled the room.

A well-dressed man came over to me and shook my hand. "Donna," he said, smiling, "I'm Doctor Dedomenico. I'm so glad you came tonight." His sincerity overwhelmed me.

Suddenly I had a feeling of belonging; my anxiety started to subside. I stammered, "Thank you," as I took a seat.

---

1. *Video available free on 20/20 LifeStyles online; see Appendix J*

I noticed that the room was filled with people just like me. I was not alone. The very first thing Dr. Dedomenico mentioned as he began to speak was that being overweight wasn't my fault. No one had ever told me that before. He said he had weighed 275 pounds and felt tremendous shame and guilt about his weight. He couldn't understand why he was excellent at his work but such a failure at controlling his weight. He said he had to be rid of that shame and guilt before he was able to successfully control his weight.

He went into detail on how our society had been conditioned by certain foods-foods that make us continually crave more foods that make us fat. Things he said completely shattered the nutrition myths I had been taught over the years. I learned how the stress and depression I'd felt about my weight had actually caused me to gain more weight. I learned about the harm I had been causing my body. I'd known I was destroying myself for a long time, but after listening to Dr. Dedomenico, I suddenly began to care about it. Maybe this time would be different.

He spoke about the body's regulatory systems and how they become chemically imbalanced when our nutrition is too high in carbohydrates. I was amazed to hear how we were capable of creating a system within ourselves that drove us to become fatter and fatter. I learned how important it is to exercise, and also how important it is to be physically active even when not exercising. I learned that the antidepressants I'd been taking for years could cause me to gain weight. I learned that my sleep problems were making me gain weight. I learned that fad diets cause you to gain weight in the long run, because they make you chemically imbalanced and place you in starvation mode. NO WONDER I WAS FAT. I HAD BEEN DOING EVERYTHING WRONG.

What really caught my attention was Dr. Dedomenico's explanation about reward-center eating and habits. I knew, at that moment, that this was why I loved sugar, fat, and salt-especially when they were combined. They triggered the feel-good chemicals in my brain-endorphins, dopamine, and serotonin. And yes, while those chemicals gave me some relief, I ultimately felt worse later. And how about those habits, my special treats, my special restaurants, and those familiar places to stop on the way home? No wonder I was addicted to food; my habits were hard-wired into my brain.

Then Dr. Dedomenico began talking about hope-the same hope I had heard on the phone when I first spoke with him. He talked about all the things we were doing wrong, and he laid out a program that addressed each and every one. The 20/20 LifeStyles program was based on many years of clinical research. It was very specific, and it made total sense to me.

Doctor Dedomenico had a team of medical doctors, psychologists, registered dietitians, and exercise physiologists who were experts in ME! There were also more than 60 educational videos and a great online app for me to use. They'd been helping people like me for 20 years and had been hugely successful. Best of all, when I talked to those experts after the seminar, they were all so kind and caring, I felt they were truly interested in me.

My desperation had actually caused me to become teachable. I trusted the 20/20 staff completely, and so, amazingly, I did everything they told me to do, just the way they told me to do it. My fear of failure was slowly replaced by growing self-confidence.

As it turned out, the miserable, depressed, and hopeless person who walked into the meeting that first night actually died. Over the course of the 20/20 LifeStyles program, a brand-new me emerged. That individual who felt shame, guilt, failure, and self-loathing no longer existed. The new me actually felt self-love and self-respect. The difference was truly staggering.

That was 4½ years ago. The bad news is, this year I turned 40. The good news is, I look 30! I ran my first half-marathon while I was in the 20/20 LifeStyles program and have run one every year since. I work out three days a week. My blood pressure is 119/72. I weigh 116 pounds, and a lot of that is muscle. My closet of tent-shaped shirts has been replaced by form-fitting dresses, and now I look and feel great! I have a new problem, though. When I go shopping, everything fits and looks great, so now I've become a clothes-horse.

I have been promoted twice, and things are still improving. You know what, I've saved the best for last. They make beautiful wedding dresses in size 4, and I just picked one out. That's right. I'm getting married in three months! THANK YOU, THANK YOU, THANK YOU, Doctor Dedomenico! You not only saved my life, you made my life precious.

When Donna accepted our invitation to attend the seminar, it required courage. It also indicated that she had taken a very important step: the first step toward a commitment for change. If you live in the Puget Sound area, you can attend this seminar for free; it may change your life just as it did Donna's. Call (425) 861-6258 for a reservation, or go online: www.2020lifestyles.com/get-started.aspx

The factors that took Donna from the depths of shame, guilt, despair and self-destruction to someone who loves her life are shown in the concepts that follow.

CONCEPT #1

If You're Overweight, You're Not Alone.

Donna felt abnormal because of her inability to lose weight. She believed she was part of a small group of people who could not manage their weight. The truth is that Donna-and you-are in the majority, because 70 percent of the population of the United States is overweight. So if you're one of those people who have been searching for the magic diet (and isn't everyone?), welcome to the unhappy majority. What's even more discouraging is the fact that less than 2 percent of people who lose a substantial amount of weight are able to maintain that weight loss. Before you throw this book at the wall and give up, please read further.

Since you've most likely tried to lose weight before, you're aware of the obstacles. For example, at times you couldn't stick to a diet and lost almost no weight, and at other times you were frustrated because your diet might have been temporarily effective but simply didn't work in the long run.

Dieting is a concern shared by about 200 million Americans, because the United States is now second only to Mexico in obesity statistics. We are an overweight nation with overweight habits and an overweight mentality that has consumed our way of life.

As designers of the 20/20 LifeStyles program, we thoroughly understand the challenges and frustrations you face, and the impact that has on your body and mind. The plain truth is this: Excess weight is killing us, shortening our lives, and making us miserable.

Yet there's plenty of room for optimism here. The message of this book is **hope.** We will take you through our method and lead you to a lifestyle that helps eliminate the health hazards of obesity and excess body fat forever.

We will teach you how to stop hating yourself and blaming yourself for your weight-loss failures, and we will introduce you to a mindset that actually allows you to love yourself and respect your body.

If you're now ready to face your weight-loss issues, weight loss can be manageable and permanent.

CONCEPT #2
Self-Blame Is Self-Destruction

People like Donna who are highly self-critical about their physical appearance are burdened by a strong sense of shame and guilt. Being overweight leads to this shame and guilt and also to feelings of being less likeable than individuals whose weight is normal. However, these feelings are completely misplaced.

Here's the simple fact: Overweight people are victims, not perpetrators. Our western culture has misled the average person with a diet that is not just unhealthy; it's also deceptive in its misrepresentation of how Americans should eat. Food manufacturers, fast-food companies, and restaurant chains constantly offer "fat-free" alternatives that are so sugar-laden they're actually fat builders. Soft drinks and other canned goods are full of high-fructose corn syrup, the food business's answer to a cheap sweetener, which actually puts on pounds while you're expecting the opposite.

Finally, the educational system in our schools and families is so misguided that food advice, if and when it occurs, is usually far off the mark.

If you're overweight, we want you to know this: **It's not your fault.** You, like so many others who've gained weight over the years, were never given the opportunity to learn or choose. Overweight people have been under attack with misinformation for decades, and the result of that assault is on display at your local doctor's office or emergency room. Our health system is swamped with health problems that our dietary faults have created: high cholesterol, high blood pressure, diabetes, coronary heart disease, and more. On your path to self-discovery, it is critical for you to accept that you must not blame yourself for your condition. If you examine your past, you will see that you were never taught to eat correctly or live a healthy lifestyle. You adopted lifelong habits and behaviors based on faulty information. Before, you never had a chance, but now you do.

CONCEPT #3

Permanent Weight Loss Takes Consistency And Patience

The urge to lose all your weight by next Tuesday (or any short time period) is self-defeating. It leads many to attempt the next new fad diet or the next new crash diet. But these diets simply reinforce our feelings of hopelessness and failure. In other words, there are no good reasons to starve yourself. That's right. Crash diets may take off a few pounds, but those who follow them haven't learned anything or changed anything in the process, and those pounds-plus some friends-inevitably return.

These diets also strengthen our misinformation about nutrition and completely miss the point about lifestyle, behavior and habit change. If you focus on your lifestyles, behaviors, and habits, not only will you reach your desired weight, you will maintain that weight.

Losing weight is not a quick or easy process. You must unlearn all the myths and wrong information you've absorbed over the years. After that, you must learn to take a sensible approach to weight management and fitness.

Not only do you have to learn about nutrition, exercise, and lifestyle change, you have to act on these changes long enough for them to become your new fixed habits. That's why it takes time. When we're under stress, new habits and behaviors collapse, and we revert to older, more familiar bad habits. It takes quite a while for your new habits to become fixed, so that they tolerate stress without collapsing.

CONCEPT #4
The Food-For-Love Replacement Cycle Leads To Unhappiness And Depression

Some of you eat because you feel unwanted, unimportant, or unloved. Like Donna, you learned at a very young age that food is love. Remember when you fell down and hurt your knee, how Mom would give you a cookie? On your birthdays you had party with pizza, cake, and ice cream. All large family gatherings and celebrations revolved around food and drink.

You learned the lesson: FOOD IS LOVE! 20, 30, or 40 years later, you're still following that model, and it hasn't worked yet!

Using this "food is love" message, you adopted a behavior pattern that became the foundation for your lack of self-esteem. You also learned that the "food as love" expression maintained by your families actually translated into a substitute for loving yourself. You misinterpreted the very real physical and emotional rewards that you felt from sugar, fat, and salt as a way to generate your own positive emotions.

The more weight you gained, the more you loathed your condition. That cycle was self-perpetuating: you would feel bad about yourself, then you'd eat foods with sugar, fat, and salt to feel better. And then you'd feel even worse about yourself. This pattern would repeat over and over again. Finally, the more often you satisfied your emotional needs with food, the more unconsciously destructive your oral reward system became.

The fact is that overweight individuals frequently have negative self-perception. Those negative feelings are a significant factor in why weight gain and obesity originally occur.

If guilt, shame, and self-loathing were an effective motivational tool against gaining weight, there would be no overweight people. Therefore, it follows that positive perceptions are essential building blocks on the road to your overall recovery.

As shown in the graphic below, the cycle begins with overeating, then come the guilt and shame, followed by eating to make yourself feel better, which augments your guilt and shame with depression. The depression causes your adrenal gland to release the hormone cortisol[2], and guess what? Cortisol makes you hungry again, which leads to weight gain, hopelessness and more eating. This self-perpetuating cycle leads to continuing depression and hopelessness. The answer to breaking this cycle is in Concept #5.

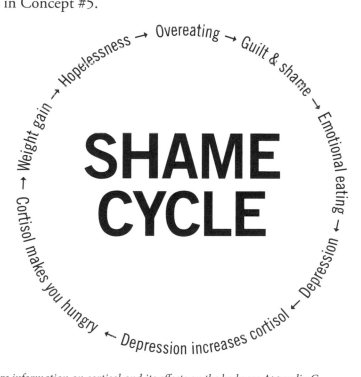

2. For more information on cortisol and its effects on the body see Appendix C.

CONCEPT #5

The Role Of Self-Respect And Self-Love Is Crucial In Health And Well-Being

The first step in achieving self-love is to resolve the guilt and the shame; that opens the door to self-acceptance.

Self-respect and self-love can only occur after self-acceptance and cannot exist at all in an individual who feels guilt or shame.

Self-acceptance to Respect your body

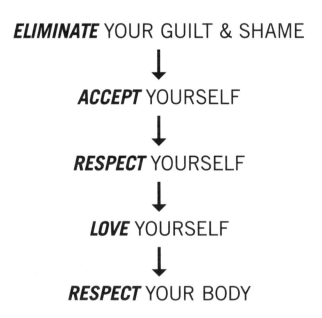

ELIMINATE YOUR GUILT & SHAME

↓

ACCEPT YOURSELF

↓

RESPECT YOURSELF

↓

LOVE YOURSELF

↓

RESPECT YOUR BODY

As you continue to read the success stories in this book, you will see that each individual had to eliminate his or her shame and guilt in order to develop self-acceptance and finally progress to self-respect and self-love.

While it's our hope that the five concepts discussed in this chapter have helped move you in that direction, by now you might be asking yourself, "How do I make the leap from self-acceptance to self-love?"

While the process is fairly easy to describe, accomplishing it can be much more difficult. To experience self-love you must "act as if." That means you have to treat yourself as if you respect and love yourself. If you do this long enough, it stops being an act and becomes you. That's a pretty simple concept, isn't it?

On the other hand, when you've just gained another five pounds and none of your clothes fit any more, or when you started your diet at 7:00 a.m. and blew it at 5:00 p.m., how do you make that self-love thing work?

Primarily, you need to understand the doctrine of unconditional acceptance something that's foreign to most of us. After all, when you break the law, you're punished. If you go against the morals of religion, you may be shunned or cast out. If you don't conform to your family's norms, you may be disowned, and so forth. You live in a society that's structured around guilt, blame, and punishment. That's all you've known throughout your life.

So how do you learn about unconditional acceptance? Where can you learn to love yourself and not feel guilty after a calorie-laden Thanksgiving dinner?

Here's the simple truth: Nobody is perfect.

We're all fallible. And although moral, legal, and ethical codes were created to form a more just and livable society, you shouldn't use them as whips and chains to punish yourself.

> *It's time you face up to it: you are and will always be fallible!*

It now becomes your goal to accept your fallibility and strive for improvement, knowing that the path will not be easy and that you will not always be successful.

> *The key to self-acceptance, self-respect, and eventually self-love is for you to accept your failures and strive to do better.*

Once you feel self-love, the world becomes a better place. You feel so good that you delight in being kind and generous to yourself. You no longer feel unworthy. You can strive for your goals without fear of failing. You begin to treat your body in a loving way, which leads to respecting your body. Once you respect your body, you can successfully lose weight, maintain your weight loss, and improve your physical condition. The result is your ability to lead a healthier, happier, and longer life.

These changes also come with an added benefit: Once you learn to love yourself, you will be amazed at the love you receive from others. This creates a new cycle that continues to support your positive changes.

CONCEPT #6
A Closed Mind Can Be Your Own Personal Prison

When you feel hopeless, you're expressing the attitude that you think you know all there is to know. You're also presuming that, based on your vast knowledge and incredible intellect, there is no solution. That line of thinking is a closed loop. There's no chance to take in new information or re-analyze your situation, and since you're closed to all new information, you're truly doomed.

Even though this closed-mindedness is terribly self-defeating, it also happens to be very comfortable. Why? Because there's no risk-no fear of new experiences, new learning, or failure. So, ironically, while closed-mindedness is a strangely comfortable prison, it is still a prison, and a deadly one.

The only way out of that prison is by forcing yourself to confront the anxiety of trying and learning new things. That breakthrough can be very uncomfortable at times. Imagine how Donna felt walking into a sports club, with the many fears in her mind. She believed that every eye in the club was on her, because she thought she didn't fit in. Worse yet, she anticipated that someone would expect her to do exercises that she couldn't do. But the worst fear of all for Donna was humiliation.

Donna had a long history of humiliations, which she relived regularly. It seemed she never forgot how badly these humiliating experiences made her feel. Her greatest fear, therefore, was not of someone else but of judging herself.

Had Donna not broken through that fear, she would most likely have quit before allowing herself to experience a very personal miracle.

So how do you prevent fear from keeping you in prison?

Well, in this case, the fear is related to two perceptions:

1. What will others think of you?
2. What you will think of yourself based on what they think of you?

Keep in mind that opinions, and especially public opinions, are often illusions.

A wise person once said, "If you get ten people to agree with you, you can form a club. If you get a thousand people to agree with you, you can form a political party, and if you get a million people to agree with you, you can form a religion." Have you ever adored some movie star, only to discover that he beats his wife? Your opinion changed instantly, didn't it? Have you admired a politician only to find out he was caught with his hand in the cookie jar? Same reversal in your perception, right? Public opinion can be deceptive and temporary. What people think of each other is fickle and changeable. If we were to take a poll in the local paper regarding opinions about you, the results would probably be something like this: 50 people like you, 50 people dislike you, and 200,000 never heard of you and frankly don't care. The point is that what counts in life is not what others think of you, but rather what you think of yourself.

What you think of yourself is the prime ingredient in self-acceptance.

You need to feel confident about turning your life around. Never have doubts about improving yourself! Remember this: You will never be doing something wrong if you're on a quest to gain knowledge about yourself, which will always make your life better. There is simply no way you can feel negative about that.

The door to self-respect and self-love is always open. It's time to come out of your prison cell and live life to the fullest.

If you haven't yet viewed the free introductory 20/20 LifeStyles videos online, you should do so at this point. Refer to Appendix J for a description of the videos and a link to them. Better yet, if you live in the Puget Sound area, attend the free introductory lecture-just call (425) 861-6258 for a reservation.

CONCEPT #7

The Hardest Part Is Starting. Then It Gets Easier

If you, like Donna, are serious about losing weight and getting healthier and have been frustrated by the yo-yo results of your previous diets, or found that your weight loss has not been complemented by an improvement in your health, then 20/20 LifeStyles is for you.

The 20/20 LifeStyles food philosophy is a result of our years of experience in the field of medical nutrition and cardiovascular research. Your plan is based on a program that has treated more than 10,000 patients with serious physical ailments, from simply being overweight to cardiac rehabilitation.

More than 20 years ago we noticed that popular high-carbohydrate/low-fat diets were not effective for overweight individuals. These diets didn't eliminate their carbohydrate cravings. Surprisingly, these diets actually stimulated hunger and cravings. That's because high-carbohydrate diets cause the release of a hormone called ghrelin[3] that makes you hungry. The green light to eat fat-free foods not only led to a diet of highly processed foods with empty calories, it also left those who followed the diet feeling less energetic, bloated, and discouraged

3. For more information on ghrelin see Appendix B.

about not losing weight. Food manufacturers today take a different approach, claiming their products promote health because they're "made with whole grains." The perception that whole grains make these foods healthful is misguided, since the products often contain only negligible amounts of whole grains. Many of those foods are high in calories, heavily processed, and have the potential to increase the risk of metabolic syndrome-also known as insulin resistance.

Virtually everyone begins our program with a body that's completely out of chemical balance. Being out of chemical balance makes you hungry. It's been our task to use medically proven methods to help you heal your body, in order to get you back into chemical balance and get yourself functioning properly in all respects.

Metabolic syndrome, or insulin resistance, carries a group of risk factors that can occur singly or in combination. Someone with metabolic syndrome has an increased risk of cardiovascular disease, stroke, type 2 diabetes, dementia, and Alzheimer's disease. A diagnosis of metabolic syndrome (insulin resistance) requires three of the following indicators:

1. Central obesity with a waist circumference greater than 35 inches for a female and 40 inches for a male.

2. Dyslipidemia*: Triglycerides greater than 150 mg/dl.

3. Dyslipidemia*: HDL (good) cholesterol less than 50 mg/dl for females and less than 40 mg/dl for males.

4. Blood pressure greater than 130/85.

5. Fasting blood sugar 118 mg/dl or more.

   * Dyslipidemia is an abnormal amount of lipids (cholesterol and/or fat) in the blood.

Certain medical conditions can contribute to metabolic syndrome. But it can also be caused by unhealthy diet, stress, inadequate sleep, aging, and central (abdominal) obesity. Central (abdominal) obesity is usually caused by an increase in visceral or intra-abdominal fat. Visceral fat cells release chemicals that cause inflammation and insulin resistance.

The average American eats more sugar in a day than our Stone Age ancestors ate in a YEAR!

Our bodies weren't designed for the present-day American diet, which we've only recently introduced. What a shock to our systems, considering that it takes hundreds of thousands of years for the human body to adapt to a new way of eating! Bear this in mind: Our Stone Age ancestors existed a mere 10,000 years ago. To put that in perspective, if we compare the history of human beings on this planet to a football field, 10,000 years would be equivalent to 6 inches. In that 6 inch span, our metabolisms have been subjected to our current American diet for too small a period to be measurable on that scale. That's how short a time we've had to adapt to this high-carbohydrate diet.

This unhealthy diet has been thrust on us by the government and the food industry, and the results are not positive. The food industry discovered that adding sugar to foods is an inexpensive way of making us eat and buy more of those foods. The result is weight gain and a cascade of metabolic disorders.

CONCEPT #8

Despite The Difficulties, There Is A Solution

The body's weight-maintenance system is very complex and fragile. Because of our society's eating habits, that system has suffered damage in a huge number of people.

As we mentioned earlier, approximately two-thirds of the people in this country are overweight. The good news is that we have a fairly good idea about how the body's weight-maintenance system works and how it gets damaged. We understand that there is a delicate balance between what we eat, what we do, and how the system functions.

The body is like a three-legged-stool. In order to function properly, all three legs must be functional. Remove one leg and the stool collapses. Those three legs are nutrition, exercise, and lifestyle.

NUTRITION

A lot of misinformation has been circulated about nutrition.

Much of that misguided data came through the food industry, which has a vested interest in getting us all to eat more. We regret to say, the medical community and the government have generated other erroneous information. That's why finding accurate nutritional information requires sorting through tons of misinformation, a job calling for diligence and expertise.

People are consuming processed grains, most of them made from refined flour as a larger proportion of their diet than the vegetables, fruits, nuts, plant oils, and lean meats we should be consuming. We noticed that many of our patients had unbalanced diets, primarily based on wheat and grain products-crackers, bagels, pastas, white rice, chips, cookies, and breads. We also found that as a result of the high consumption of these foods their metabolism was out of balance. This imbalance caused hunger cravings, unhealthy blood-sugar levels, vulnerability to inflammation, and elevated stress hormones including cortisol.

It may sound more familiar if we tell you that this is why you weren't losing weight or are even gaining it, especially around your waist.

You see, these extra pounds around your abdomen, known as visceral abdominal fat, are unlike any fat stored elsewhere in your body. Visceral abdominal fat triggers a metabolic cascade of health risks. We discuss visceral abdominal fat at greater length in the introductory videos and also in Chapter 7, Concept #20.

In addition to the carbohydrates mentioned above, the public rarely hears mention of sugar substitutes. These are such artificial sweeteners as aspartame, saccharin, stevia, sucralose, and the rest. Even though these supposedly "sugar-free"" sweeteners are marketed as diet aids, they actually cause you to gain weight. That's right. They cause you to gain weight!

Aspartame, discovered in 1965, was predicted to dramatically decrease our society's sugar consumption. In 1965, Americans consumed about 75 pounds of sugar and corn sweetener (high-fructose corn syrup) per person per year[4] and an estimated one pound of artificial sweetener per year. Last year, the average American consumed about 190 pounds of various sugars[5] and corn sweetener per year and an estimated 26 pounds[6] of artificial sweeteners. So, as you see, artificial sweeteners had the opposite effect on sugar consumption, and it's our guess that you probably went with the trend and are likely above average.

Additionally, as Americans increased their consumption of high-fructose corn syrup[7], sugar, and artificial sweeteners, they also decreased their consumption of both healthy fats and protein, with the result that they get hungrier and get hungry more often.

Many of you who crave sweets or grain-based products have experienced their addictive quality during the withdrawal from these foods. Processed grain and other such wheat products as cookies,

4. Source U.S. Dept. of Agriculture.
5. These include fructose, lactose, maltose, and dextrose.
6. As of 1987 the government no longer collects data on artificial-sweetener consumption.
7. More on high-fructose corn syrup in Chapter 8, Concept #22.

pretzels, crackers, chips, muffins, etc., break down into simple sugars as soon as you eat them. They often stimulate hunger and a strong urge to eat more of them [8].

Symptoms of withdrawal from grain and carbohydrate foods can include cravings for sweets or starchy grain products, fatigue, mental fogginess, depression, and irritability. Fortunately, we have found that this phase lasts only about three to four days after the elimination of simple carbohydrates in Stage 1 of the meal plan [9].

Modern wheat has undergone genetic changes over the past 50 years, mostly to provide a greater yield per acre. These changes have altered the gluten protein structure, a change that can cause immune responses in many individuals. These immune responses result in a series of metabolic complications ranging from mild rashes, bloating, and difficulty losing weight, to more serious digestive complications leading to celiac disease. Celiac disease, caused by dietary wheat intolerance, is on the rise, having increased fourfold over the past 50 years.

Your diet has to conform to your body's chemistry. Although everyone's body chemistry is different and individual people have different tolerances to grains, there are some general nutritional rules. As you will see in later chapters, we use an elimination diet that meets these nutritional needs but tailors the plan for each individual's body chemistry.

EXERCISE

Exercise is another area awash with false information. Exercise must also be individualized for each person based on condition, purpose, and time constraints. Remember that the latest fad in exercise is often just as damaging as the latest fad diet. Our 20/20 LifeStyles physical therapists have seen the harm caused by exercise fads. The best

8. For more information, see Nutrition videos Carbs and Sugar, in Appendix J.
9. See Stage 1 meal plan in Chapter 9.

personalized exercise program requires an assessment of each individual's lifestyle, health, capabilities, fitness level, and past levels of fitness. We will create an exercise program for you in Chapter 9.

LIFESTYLE

A good deal of research has been done on the effects of genetics on longevity, but no strong correlations have been found. That's because, as our own experience tells us, lifestyles, behaviors, and habits have a much greater effect on longevity than genetics. Here's the good news: Since lifestyles are learned, they can be relearned. Doing so takes serious effort, however-an investment of time and a commitment to consistency.

Medical knowledge is available to address problems with nutrition, exercise, and lifestyle. Over the last 25 years we've organized what we've learned into a successful step-by-step plan for repairing broken metabolic systems. That information is the focus of this book.

In the following chapters, you'll find information from our dietitians, exercise physiologists, and counselors that will teach you how to be successful and stay successful at each stage of our plan.

If you fully embrace the need for a lifestyle change, the results will be amazing to you and those you know. Besides Donna's story, this book contains many stories recounting how people like you found a road to a better life, using the guidance we gave them along the way. Also, we would very much like to hear your stories. Please send us your stories, your successes, and your challenges. Send them to us at lifestylesbook@proclub.com.

CHAPTER 2

BUILDING YOUR SUPPORT SYSTEM

SOMETIMES COURAGE HAS A QUIET VOICE
Diana, age 42

My change actually started one night when my husband and I were sitting in the living room and it hit me like a brick. It was well after dinner, and my three kids were off in their rooms getting ready for bed, when I looked across at my husband. Here I was, sipping a beer, doing what he expected, drinking because he was drinking. It seemed we couldn't have a conversation any more unless we had a drink in our hands. I looked across at him and saw him through new eyes-my drunken husband with his belly hanging out, grazing on potato chips as he watched sports on TV.

I remember wondering why I treated him with so much consideration when he treated me so badly.

In that moment my life came into focus. I realized that from the time when I was a young girl, I hadn't been satisfied unless I was working hard to please those around me, particularly men. Then I had another alarming thought: Nothing about my tendency for servitude would ever change.

As I sat in my chair, that thought really began to frighten me. Contemplating the worst, I became more anxious. I was so jumpy I couldn't sit still. I shifted my weight repeatedly, but my husband was oblivious as usual, and as the minutes passed I worked up the courage to say something.

"You know," I ventured, "I think I need a change."

"Huh?" He continued to stare at the screen.

"I said, I need to change my life."

"That's nice, honey."

Irritated, I said, "You're not listening to me."

When I finally got his attention, I told him I wanted a chance to do something different about myself. I was too fat and I knew it. What I couldn't tell him was that I was tired of trying to keep up with his alcoholic habits. Drinking had dominated our lives and caused frequent duress for me and the kids.

I explained to my husband that I wanted to try a different lifestyle, and that meant signing up for the 20/20 LifeStyles program.

He looked at me like I was crazy.

"Ah, you're over-reacting to a bad day," he said. "You're just tired; you'll feel better in the morning."

When I insisted I was going to sign up, he must have felt threatened, because then he got scary mad.

"What will I do with myself," he demanded, "with you away from home doing those sessions?"

"I can make it work," I said. "We'll have our time together."

He wasn't satisfied. "And what about the money? How d'you plan to pay for the program?"

"I'll take it out of my savings. That's my own money. I should be able to do what I want with it."

He had always complained angrily when I wanted to do anything outside the home.

"You have enough responsibilities right here," he went on. "Why are you trying to make my life difficult?"

I showed him the courtesy of hearing him out, but when I still insisted I wanted to join the program, he got really suspicious.

"Why are you suddenly so willing to spend time away from home?" He squinted at me and popped open another beer. "Trying to find an excuse? You having an affair or something?"

I scoffed. "You know that's ridiculous." Nearly 50 pounds overweight, I couldn't imagine being attractive to anyone. "I just want to be beautiful again. I need to change."

"There's nothing wrong with the way you are." He took a foamy swallow. "Besides, you're beautiful to me, and that's all that counts."

I sat there staring at him. I knew I'd hit a brick wall. My willingness to cater to my husband's wishes and give in to him had brought me to this juncture in my life. It took hold in my brain: He was an alcoholic, and to please him, I had become one too.

By trying to keep peace, what I called my "life" was filled with domestic activity-none of it devoted to my needs. I never took time for myself. I had a full-time job, three kids whom I cared for when I wasn't working, and a demanding man who had to have everything his way.

My day would begin at 5:00 a.m. I would hustle to get the kids off to school, prepare breakfast for the family, get dressed, and be at work by 8:30 a.m.. Then, after work, because it was part of the ritual, I would meet my husband at our favorite bar for several drinks at happy hour and dinner. Sometimes he'd hang out there for more drinks, or sometimes he'd come home with me, but either way I would rush back to the house to feed my brood, ages 9, 16, and 18, by 6:00 p.m., then do the rest of the kitchen clean-up and other housekeeping for the rest of the evening. And the next day it started all over again.

We had a horrible argument that evening, all because I was ready to try to do something positive for myself. I was scared and confused, but after a lot of soul searching and putting it off a couple of days, I finally called 20/20 LifeStyles. I went there on my lunch break, and as I enrolled, I knew full well that my husband was going to be very upset.

That's when the status quo in our marriage ended. I hung in there, trying to fit my husband's alcoholic lifestyle, even while I was trying new meal plans and exercise. It was brutal, because any progress I made physically was neutralized by having to drink cocktails every evening to keep the peace.

In the meantime, the counseling I got at the clinic helped me understand why I had evolved into a male-dominated woman. Recounting my history in my counseling sessions revealed a lot. For one thing, my mom left my dad when I was four, and although I saw her on occasion, she really wasn't an influence in my life. My dad was a workaholic and, perhaps because his wife had deserted him, very hypercritical of me as a female. Nothing I did was good enough, and I felt inferior. Dad was especially disappointed in my lack of athletic ability, and dissatisfied with anything but perfect grades. I tried so hard to get top grades, because it was the only way to get any positive attention from him.

Somehow my willingness to please men continued right into puberty, and I needed male company at a very early age. Those girl-boy relationships were in keeping with my childhood. I needed approval from my boyfriends, just as I had from my father. The way I would achieve approval, by the way, was to find dysfunctional young men who depended on me for a number of things they couldn't or wouldn't do for themselves. In fact, they were so dysfunctional that my mom, whom I still saw occasionally, was judgmental and called me a "bum magnet." It was true. Every one of my boyfriends she ever met was a moocher.

43

The day my male bondage ended was the day I signed up for 20/20 LifeStyles and defied my husband. After that, everything rotated 180 degrees. Where my identity had revolved around my husband's approval, the life lessons I learned convinced me I was finally, and for the first time, my own person in charge of my life. I verbalized that to my lifestyle counselors, and I could say it with pride: "I, alone, am responsible for the quality of my life."

It was the statement that defined my complete departure from male dependency.

The combination of dietary guidance, exercise, and counseling did wonders. Before, I would always overeat the wrong foods, because I allowed myself to get too hungry. Now I was meal tracking and keeping my calorie counts in line. The exercise routines were built for me specifically, and the lifestyle counseling-well, the counseling helped me to see the world totally differently.

I came to realize I had a great degree of stress in my home and how I was distraught due to the chaos created by the alcoholic culture of my marriage. As my eyes began to open, I could see my utter lack of self-respect. I had allowed others to discount my own feelings in any decision-making, and I was afraid to stand up for myself. I had been a mindless eater, putting anything into my mouth without even tasting or enjoying it. Now I recognized that what I put in my mouth was fuel for my body and my mind. I was beginning to respect myself and respect my body.

Finally, the team at 20/20 became the support group I didn't have at home. They became my friends-friends who changed my life. A crucial moment came when I was talking to my personal Lifestyle Counselor and Dr. Mark Dedomenico, the founder of the program, about how hard it was for me to quit drinking because my husband expected me to drink with him.

Doctor Dedomenico listened carefully, then put an arm around me and told me he wanted to make a deal. He said that if I would quit alcohol, he would gift the rest of the program to me just so I could finish. The generosity of that offer did it. I never looked back. I was going to finish, even if it cost me my marriage.

It was the most important decision of my life, and it meant everything. I went on to lose 48½ pounds. I totally changed the shape of my body. I divorced my husband. I became a new person, and I mean that statement literally. My old habits, my old feelings, and my old dependency died that day when I came alive. No longer was I pleasing everyone else at my own expense. I was taking care of me.

I had always thought of my weight, my marriage, and my drinking as things I had to live with. But I know now that I can accomplish anything if I want it badly enough. I'm so full of positive energy right now, I feel like conquering a lot of other mountains in my life.

In fact, I have plans to climb Mount St. Helens this summer. If you want to join me, I'll race you to the top!

CONCEPT #9
I Can't Do It... But We can!

Diana clearly didn't have support in her home for the changes she desperately wanted to make. In fact, she lived in a system that made change all but impossible.

Some of you have wonderful built-in support systems in your home, immediate family, and extended family. Others have excellent support systems with your friends. But many of you have inadequate support systems. While lack of close friends and family can be a challenge, the worst-case scenarios are situations where individuals have a tear-down system rather than a support system. Tear-down people are those who need to control others, and believe their only way to control you is to make you feel small, insignificant, unworthy, and unattractive. These destructive individuals feel secure only when you feel miserable and insecure.

Unfortunately for Diana, she was living in a tear-down system.

We hope this isn't your circumstance. You must find support to make your plan work from Day One and for the rest of your life. Having support is part of a successful weight-loss plan and, more importantly, part of successfully maintaining that weight loss.

If you're married, gaining support from your spouse from Day One is ideal. Many of our patients have spouses who attend dietitian and lifestyle counselor sessions with them, eat with them, and work out with them. To get support from your spouse, though, you have to open up the communication channels. You have to sit down and explain your weight and/or metabolic disorder, then discuss exactly how you plan to deal with it.

This means you have to let go of the guilt and shame related to your weight and/or metabolic disorder. You need to honestly tell your spouse that you need his or her help, and what form you would like that help to take. This is doubly important if you have children living in your home. In fact, if the children are old enough, explain it to them and ask for their support. You may be helping them build healthy habits too.

Be specific with what you need from everyone in your support system. If you want them to help you with your nutrition, then review the steps of the meal plan with them. If you want them to exercise or go walking with you, let them know what days and what times you need them. Depending on how receptive your spouse is to your discussion, you can suggest that he or she read this book. In explaining just what kind of support you need, make sure you're clear about what you do and don't want.

For instance, tell your spouse not to hide food from you. Say that if you find it, you'll feel resentful. Explain which foods should be eliminated from the house, so you won't be so likely to slip when you get cravings or have a weak moment. Besides, eliminating these foods from the house is healthy for the whole family. Tell them because this is a journey, not to expect perfection. Weight and metabolic problems are chronic disorders that are difficult to overcome. Explain that you may have slips, or what we call lapses, along the way, but you'll recover and learn from those slips. Ask them not to police, lecture, criticize, or reprimand you. It doesn't make the situation any better, and if you feel judged, that can make it worse.

They can do several things to help you succeed on this plan, for example, keep a positive attitude through the good times and especially through the frustrating times. Find time during the week to talk with your support team about how the plan is going and how this book is changing your thinking about nutrition and exercise.

Have a discussion with your family or your housemates, and tell them that in the early stages of your plan, it is not recommended for you to entertain, dine out, or travel. Together, you will need to develop new activities and interests that involve less food and more physical activity. This could be a major lifestyle change for all of you. Lastly, ask them to keep an open mind about trying new healthier foods and restaurants, because your eating habits are definitely going to change.

Understand that this may not always be easy. If it were, you'd have a sainted spouse and children, or roommates who didn't complain a bit about their anxieties. And, let's face it, getting all the junk food out of the house or office may be a hardship, because eating it will be less convenient for those you live or work with. Eating at fast-food restaurants less often might also seem a deprivation. Be sensitive to their needs as well, and suggest where and how they can have their special treats. Suggest some fun activities they might enjoy that are active rather than passive. Make it work well for them, so it can work well for you.

Now, what do you do if you live alone, you're not married, or your spouse isn't supportive? Who will support you? Certainly other family members can be part of your team, but it would be better to find someone who's trying to overcome the same weight and/or metabolic disorder you are-or even better, someone who has successfully lost weight and kept it off. There are many more people around than you may think.

If being overweight is the metabolic disorder you're trying to overcome, don't expect friends who've never had a weight problem to understand what it's like to be driven to eat half a cheesecake because you're out of chemical balance. They've obviously never felt the same drives, cravings, and desires that you have. They've also never felt the out-of-control feelings or the shame and guilt.

> *Most people whose weight is normal don't understand that:*
>
> > - *Our bodies have set points* which cause them to resist weight loss.*
> >
> > - *We've tried many diets and failed, resulting in low self-esteem, hopelessness, and feelings of failure.*
> >
> > - *Like an alcoholic, we respond to chemical pulls and can fall off the wagon at any time, but we can also use these lapses as learning experiences.*
> >
> > - *Certain foods make us chemically out of balance, causing us to think about and look for food. People who don't have this problem eat those foods*

without getting out of chemical balance and hungry.

- *A stressful situation can make us hungry, while the same stressful situation will make them stop eating.*

- *Our brain cells have long memories of how good certain foods taste, or how those foods will comfort us through our reward center, when we are stressed or depressed.*

- *Overweight people are usually very sensitive. They would rather be care-givers than care-receivers. It's very difficult to accept help from others, and even harder to put ourselves first.*

   * *Your body's biological set point resists changes in your weight. Resetting it can be difficult.*

Knowing the points listed above will allow you to understand why people whose weight is normal can be part of your support group, but not your key supporters. So, whom will you look to as a key supporter? The best person is someone who has lost weight on a food plan, or is losing weight on a food plan successfully.

After you find a compatible support partner, mentor, or workout buddy, you'll find having a partner makes it easier to exercise even on those days when you don't feel like it. And after you finish your plan, the two of you can continue to exercise and discuss your nutrition plans and challenges. You can train together toward some event such as a 5K race, climbing a nearby mountain, going on a long bike ride, or some other activity. Your workout will now become more than just exercise. It will become educational and social, as you exchange ideas on nutrition, meal tracking, exercise, and lifestyle. And it will be fun.

We've found that many support partners do other activities together. They share recipes, go shopping, take weekend hikes or bike rides, and dine out together. And keep in mind, support partnerships work for both men and women. In most instances, we have found that it works best when your support person is of your same sex.

After you and your support partner have been together for a while, you might reach out and help another person.

So make one of your immediate priorities to start surrounding yourself with a great support team. Find at least one person who can be your key support person for exercise and continued education. And, as soon as you and your partner are able, reach out and help another person who is trying to lose weight or correct a metabolic disorder[10].

If you can't seem to find a good support partner, it might be best to get the help of a counselor who is knowledgeable about the difficulties involved in weight loss and weight maintenance, or, if you live in the Puget Sound area, contact one of our counselors: www.proclub.com/Wellness/Counseling

Support, not food, is an honest way of showing love and respect. Partnerships are one more way for you to feel good about your health, your life, and yourself.

10. For more information, see Finding Support video in LifeStyle Series videos, Appendix J.

CONCEPT #10

I Know What You Need, But I Don't Know What I Need

You may have heard the clinical term "codependency."

This word describes why Diana was so focused on pleasing others that she couldn't even consider pleasing herself. Is this like you? Do you oscillate between submission and anger and often find the anger directed at yourself? Unfortunately, some codependent individuals learn that they can literally stuff down the anger with food. Have you ever done that?

Codependents are usually created at a very early age. They're taught that everyone else's feelings are more important than their own. They're also taught that it's rude to express their true feelings and to ever say no. They're criticized whenever their behavior is not exactly the way their elders expect, even when those expectations have never been stated.

Codependents feel they can do nothing right. They feel totally unworthy and believe they have no right to feel anything. They are the Mr. or Mrs. Fixits. They try to fix everything in their family, their workplace, or social group. When these attempts at social management fail, as they usually do, the codependent person feels angry and even more useless.

Obviously, codependence is not a happy mental place. Many of the patients we see in our program are codependents, like Diana. They have focused their lives outward, never considering their own needs. They eat excessively in reaction to their disappointments and unhappiness, and since that unhappiness is ongoing, they continue to eat.

For many of these people, the 20/20 LifeStyles program was the first time they'd ever really done anything for themselves. Luckily, unlike Diana, the vast majority don't get divorced, but they do have to rearrange the power structure in their family or social group.

Power doesn't have to be 50/50 to be acceptable, but it can't be 90/10 either. Every one of us needs to get at least some of our needs met. We also need to have some input into decisions that affect our lives. We can't give "it" all to others; we need to have some of "it" for ourselves.

Our counselors spend a great deal of time talking about considerate assertiveness and how to manage your life and time in a manner that allows you to be a full person. Assertive techniques are simple, but knowing when, where, and how to use them and having the courage to do so is much, much harder. Still, with education and support it becomes quite possible.

If codependence is an issue for you, we highly recommend that you read Codependent No More, by Melody Beattie and work through the Codependent No More Workbook exercises.

CONCEPT #11
I Get No Respect!

"I get no respect!" That's a one-liner from a famous comedian, but the subject of respect, and especially self-respect, is very serious. It caused Diana to be unhappy for many years.

> *We've talked extensively about self-love in this book. We've also described how loving yourself is essential for positive self-change, so ask yourself: Can you love yourself if you don't first have self-respect?*

We have also described how self-acceptance is necessary to achieve self-love. But self-acceptance alone is not enough. It is possible to have self-acceptance without self-respect. You can accept "who you are," even though you believe that "who you are" is not worthy of respect. In other words, you can accept that you are not worthy or likeable. But if that's the kind of self-acceptance you have, can you have self-love without having self-respect? We don't believe that's possible. Self-respect is a necessary precursor to self-love.

To achieve self-respect, you must recognize your value in the world, along with your value to family, friends, employer, and others in your environment. And, most of all, you must recognize your value to yourself. This can only happen if you treat yourself with respect.

So how do you treat yourself with respect? We mentioned earlier about forgiving yourself when you've made a mistake or haven't succeeded at a goal. But it's more than that. It's also recognizing the ways you please yourself: taking the time to relax or enjoy something, getting a massage, having a night out with friends or family, and many, many other things.

Most importantly, self-respect comes from respecting your body.

One way or another, your body (and your mind, which is part of your body) gives you great service and joy. Treating another person with respect means you show them appreciation and kindness. Abusing others is definitely not a sign of respect; it's a sign of disrespect.

Abusing your body is definitely not a sign of respect.

So, in order to love yourself, you MUST treat your body with respect and not with abuse. It's clearly disrespectful to eat and drink foods that have been proven to harm your body. Not getting the proper amount of exercise is disrespectful. Not having adequate sleep, having excess stress, not having necessary medical treatment, and not taking time to relax fall into the same category of disrespect.

> *Without self-respect you cannot have self-love, and without self-love you will not respect your body and cannot be successful in maintaining a healthy weight.*

We know some of you are saying "Wow, that's a tall order," and we agree. So now you have the answer to why you have failed at diets. Being successful at maintaining weight loss means changing your lifestyle. Without that, it's just another diet.

> *In this book we will tell you what to eat and when and how to exercise. But make no mistake, without changes in your lifestyle behavior and habits; you will NOT have long-term success.*

CONCEPT #12
You Need A Healthy Body To Have A Healthy Mind

Diana felt inadequate because she couldn't please her father by excelling at sports. Her body had let her down, so she focused on using her mind and excelled at school. Like most of you, Diana felt that her body and her mind were totally different systems. But your brain is part of your body, and the nutrition that you feed your body also feeds your brain. Many of you may feel the same way: You can excuse your body for its poor performance, but you pride yourself on your mind. You like to feel in control of your emotions, to feel intelligent, to be able to carry on rewarding conversations with others, and to feel as if you're in control of your behavior.

The last few years have seen a body of research emerge on how damaging poor nutritional habits are to our brain and our mind. Research on children has shown that diets high in simple carbohydrates and sugars cause aggression, hyperactivity, and other mental-health issues[11]. A diet high in fat, especially saturated fat, and sugar damages proteins called neurotrophins, which protect the brain and help it to grow new brain cells. Sugar and fat also diminish your brain's capacity to deal with stress and depression. Research also shows that fat consumption increases the risk of depression, decreases cognitive functioning (reasoning, planning, and general intelligence), disrupts memory function, and increases the risk of dementia and Alzheimer's disease[12]. And, recent studies show that diets high in non-natural sugars (such as high-fructose corn syrup) are linked to brain dysfunction, further affecting memory and general cognition[13].

A study of 6,500 British civil servants showed that cognitive impairment in aging, overweight, and obese individuals occurred 22.5 percent faster than in individuals of normal weight[14].

Diets high in fat, sugar, refined grains, simple carbohydrates, and non-natural sugars are linked to a plethora of brain dysfunctions, including stress, depression, cognitive impairment, memory problems, dementia, and Alzheimer's disease.

You can't have a healthy mind without a healthy body.

11. *PLOS ONE, September 21, 2011; J Am Acad Child Adolesc Psychiatry, August 2013.*
12. *Ann Neurol, 2012;72; JAMA Neurol June 17, 2013.*
13. *Nutr J, 2013;12.*
14. *Whitehall II Prospective Cohort Study.*

As you can see from these studies, unhealthy eating not only damages your body, it also damages your mind. To make the problem even more disturbing, you don't know it's happening.

When you have a problem with your body, you usually feel bad. Maybe activity is hard for you, you get winded easily, you have headaches or muscle aches, or you have pain. The problem with damage to your mind is that it happens very slowly, and since it's happening to your mind, you can't detect it. Basically, you lose your intellect and your memories and start down the road to dementia and Alzheimer's disease.

Healthy foods and exercise increase the production of chemicals in your brain that make you smarter and able to think more clearly and improve your memory.

As you read this book, you will see that the 20/20 LifeStyles plan is designed to give you both a healthy body and a healthy mind.

CHAPTER 3

FINDING THE COURAGE
TO CHANGE

IN THE MIRROR, I SAW A FAILURE
Renee, age 42

From my earliest years, I felt I was a disappointment to my parents. My disposition was ruled by the idea that no matter what I did or how hard I tried, it wasn't good enough and never would be. That's how my life began, with low self-esteem and negative self-talk.

Even when I was in preschool my parents were judgmental and critical of me. They either ignored me or were annoyed by me. I felt they would be much happier if I weren't around at all. Instead of being a valued member of the family, I felt more like an accident of nature, one they were forced to deal with.

I worked tirelessly to please them and focused my attention on my studies. I thought this could be a way to get positive attention from my parents. As it turned out, my grades were excellent, yet despite my efforts their disapproval never changed. Most often you are what your parents teach you to be, and they taught me that I was singularly unlovable and unlikable. So it was only natural that by the time I became a teenager, I truly hated myself.

As I grew older, I continued to be extremely hard on myself, demanding perfection in many areas of my life. I hoped that by being perfect I might finally be good enough. Constant fear of failure also made me a paranoid control freak. I was so concerned about my image and how others perceived me that I would try to dictate everything around me in hopes that I might somehow have a chance to excel. Deep down, I always knew these efforts would end in failure.

How about that for a paradox? It was pathetic, now that I look back on it.

I would put controls in place to give myself assurances. I would accept a challenge even when convinced I would fail, and then I would manufacture ways to ruin my efforts. That cycle of doom became my expectation, that no matter what I did, or how hard I tried, it would never work.

My defeatist attitude also made me a vulnerable partner. When I had boyfriends, I would consider myself unworthy of them and lucky to have any relationship at all. Those feelings of inferiority led to a 7-year relationship with a man who enjoyed abusing me. Because of my lack of self-respect, I allowed the abuse to go on. I was addicted to him in a kind of mental masochism.

My self-esteem was so desperately low that I didn't care about myself or the way I looked. I gained weight largely because I didn't care what I ate or what it did to me. Food was my only comfort in life. It was my only friend, and it didn't judge me. I enjoyed eating fatty foods with abandon. That indulgence provided a sort of relief from pain and stress, and because I came from a Hispanic family, holidays and other family celebrations were caloric orgies in which I gladly immersed myself.

Oddly, while struggling through all my self-criticism, I still tried to achieve some objectives. This was, I suppose, part of my perfectionism and deep-seated need to excel at something. Somehow, my control-freak leanings were in a constant battle with my belief in predestined failure, and in that fight, on occasion the perfectionist, the anal-retentive side of me actually won out. For example, I worked hard enough to get a job at a prominent software company. I also earned an MBA and, much to my surprise, I found a man who would marry me. Even with all that, as the years passed, I was still totally miserable.

By that time I had sought psychiatric help, which had some effect on my mental housecleaning. But I must tell you that even while I made some headway, the doldrums would always return, bringing with them gloom and depression.

But it wasn't until I joined 20/20 LifeStyles that, with their help and love, I was able to reinvent myself.

I've been asked why and how a person with my negative attitude could even try to improve. The fact is, I entered the program convinced that it would lead nowhere, and I would fail yet again. I considered it a waste of time.

By some accident I had met and married a really nice man, and I would never have signed up if it weren't for his encouragement.

To my surprise, the staff at 20/20 were so immediately supportive, caring, genuine, devoted, and dedicated to my success that even my stubborn negativity started to change. As I discovered, their M.O., which was incredibly genuine, was that they would love me until I could love myself.

It wasn't one of those programs where they rip you down to get to the roots of your problems and then build you up again. On the contrary, from Day One, I realized that they were designing every routine, every piece of advice, specifically for my needs. Slowly, I really came to believe that it might be possible for me to change, and realizing that, something remarkable had happened. For the very first time in my life, I actually let go!

I let go of the misery, the self-hatred, and the failure. There was so much warmth and true human friendship in that organization that I decided to let the experts do their work. Can you imagine? Me, a control freak, allowing these people to tell me what I should do to help myself!

The key was my being able to trust them completely, which I did, and the results were quite amazing. I lost 23 pounds. I got into great shape. I am tight, muscle-toned, and leaner than I have ever been in my life, and in doing so, I've gained an incredible degree of self-confidence.

You know what else I got? A sense of humor.

I can now look back at my sorry existence prior to my life change, and I can laugh.

When it comes to food, I learned to incorporate it into my life as part of a healthy balance. In the past, everything about eating was good or bad. 20/20 LifeStyles demonstrated that I could attain what they call a self-slimming mindset, which means that you get so comfortable with your new knowledge and health that you automatically make the right choices without having to think about it.

So, how do I feel about my life right now? I'm in the best physical shape I've ever been in. I've gained a better balance between my expectations and the possible outcomes. And, as part of the self-slimming mindset, I've learned to allow myself to automatically and reliably choose a responsible way to conduct my life.

You see, I actually enjoy taking care of myself-and that's because I'm actually quite fond of the person I've become.

Renee was instilled with a self-defeating attitude in childhood. That attitude kept her locked in place. She "knew" she was a failure, so she continued to live in that role.

CONCEPT #13

Don't Look Back On Past Performance

Like Renee, many of you have felt like diet disasters. You have failed repeatedly at multiple diets. When you did lose weight, you started gaining it back before long, and the only benefit you got from the diet was an additional 5-pound bonus that set your weight even higher than before you started. Who wouldn't feel discouraged and depressed? Who wouldn't feel like a failure?

DIETS DON'T WORK

That's because diets don't work! That's right, we'll say it again.

As we mentioned earlier, less than 2 percent of those who lose a substantial amount of weight are able to maintain that weight loss. If you're reading this book because you're looking for the next new diet, stop reading. On the other hand, if you're convinced you need a lifestyle change to accomplish your weight and health goals-read on-because we will show you how to do that.

As we've said, your diet has to be specific to your body chemistry, and everyone's body chemistry is different.

There is one primary factor you'll need to succeed in your lifestyle change. It's important, as you start our plan, for you to keep an open mind. Don't look back at your previous failures and say, "Oh, I've tried that, it doesn't work." If you do that, you'll be beaten before you've begun. Again, it's important that you read this book with an open mind and follow our suggestions. We've helped many thousands of people lose weight and keep it off. We've also helped them achieve ultimate health and happiness. So, even though you may have failed many times before, if you focus on your goals and follow our plan, you will succeed.

That's why we've included personal stories of our past patients. As you read through the stories, you'll probably find one that sounds like you. These stories were meant for you to understand that if these people could succeed at reaching their goals, you certainly can as well. You should also understand that we have never had a person in our program who hadn't experienced previous failures. You are not alone, so keep an open mind and don't look back.

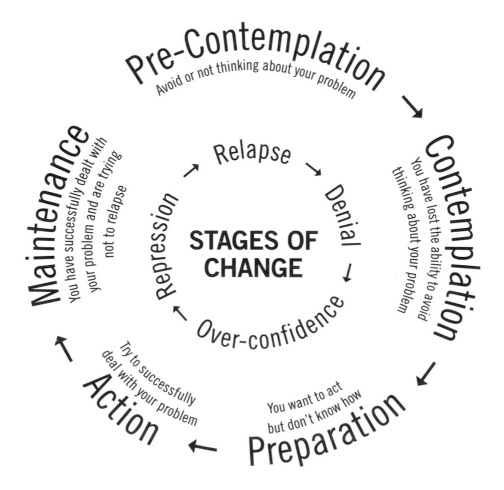

In the chart to the left, the outer circle describes how we make positive changes; the inner circle describes what happens when we relapse.

Let's describe in detail how you make the changes to achieve this new mindset. You begin with *pre-contemplation.*

Pre-contemplation is where you were before you decided to read this book.

You ate when and what you wanted. You spent considerable energy avoiding thoughts of what you were doing to your body. You rationalized, denied, or simply avoided looking at the issue completely. You just didn't want to deal with it.

Then, along the way, something happened to you. It could have been like Donna's disastrous date in Chapter 1, or Diana's insights about her husband in Chapter 2, or a doctor's diagnosis-or maybe it was you simply looking at yourself in the mirror. Whatever it was that stimulated your realization that you needed a change, you knew you couldn't avoid the issue any longer, but you also knew, or thought you knew, you could do nothing about it. After all, you had tried many times and failed.

When that realization took hold, you had moved into the *contemplation stage.* You accepted that there was a problem, but you just couldn't find the motivation to try again.

At that point, you realized you could only live with misery for so long. And when you finally couldn't stand it any longer, you made a decision to do something about it. You didn't know what you were going to do, but you had made up your mind to do something. That's when you moved into the *preparation stage.*

In the *preparation stage,* you started looking for a path to make yourself feel better physically and emotionally. And then you found this book. Perhaps you've gotten this book and, having read it to this point, you can relate to the content, but you haven't yet begun the plan.

Remember, in the Introduction we told you to begin the food plan whenever you were ready. We hope that what you've read so far has propelled you into the *action stage,* and you've started Stage 1 (Chapter 9) of the 20/20 LifeStyles plan.

If so, congratulations! You are now committed and focused on the goal of losing weight, getting in shape, and being healthy. This has become a real priority for you-and we define a priority on the basis of time, energy, and money spent on something. Simply saying, "Yes, this is a priority" without investing in it takes you back into denial and the pre-contemplative stage(15).

> *You've now seen how you went from pre-contemplation (where you were before you addressed your problem), to contemplation (where you acknowledged the problem but didn't commit to doing anything yet), to the preparation stage (where you made up your mind to do something but didn't know what exactly), to the action stage (where you committed to a plan) and, the last stage is maintenance. Maintenance will be a topic that we cover at length in Chapter 13.*

15. JO Prochaska, JC Norcross, CC DiClemente, *Changing for Good: A Revolutionary Six-Stage Program for Overcoming Bad Habits and Moving Your Life Positively Forward (New York: W. Morrow, 1994).*

CHAPTER 4

TAKING CONTROL

MY BRAIN KEPT SCREAMING FOR FOOD
Rage, age 45

Yes, Rage is really my name, but I am and always have been an easy-going person. One of the most frustrating things in my life was sticking to a behavior pattern, when I had no idea of why I was doing it.

When I look back on my youth, that's how it was for me. I was in an eating frenzy without understanding why.

Admittedly, my dad and mom were heavy, and undoubtedly they established my early dietary patterns.

As a child, I remember drinking sodas like they were water and just inhaling all kinds of sugars and carbohydrates. Of course, I knew I was a heavy kid, and I tried to correct that. I tried dieting for the first time when I was nine years old, but I failed and failed again and again. This left me accepting my ravenous relationship with food as part of my personality and my life.

The only time I was truly weight conscious occurred when I tried to get in shape for sports. Any concerns I had for my weight soon passed after I graduated from high school. When I joined the stress-filled work force, I fell into the cycle of using food as a tranquilizer for a tough day and a reward system for getting my work done. When I took breaks at work, I would slam down something sweet or fatty, and when I got home, I'd raid the refrigerator for the duration of the evening.

I got married at 24 to someone who had the same eating behaviors as me. My wife and I were basically binge buddies. The fact that she was prone to being overweight like me made it easier for both of us to ignore our nutrition and weight issues, since we knowingly overindulged together.

By the time I reached the age of 36, I weighed around 250 pounds and was still gaining weight. I had fallen into a mindset that I now equate with alcoholism: I was fully immersed in my addiction to food yet in complete denial about it being a problem. In fact, when I looked in the mirror, I didn't see an overweight guy standing there.

Much of that changed when I had to have surgery. They replaced a valve in my heart that was faulty because of a genetic flaw. But my doctors were alarmed at my weight and strongly advised me to do something about it. In their estimation, I was in really bad health, and if I didn't make changes, I would be in even deeper trouble. I believed their concerns were well founded, because I truly felt horrible. I was in a lot of physical pain, morbidly obese, and depressed most of the time. As a result, I was socially withdrawn and, because of my pain and depression, my mood swings were very tough on my family.

I realize now that I was mentally abusing my wife and children without even knowing it. Just like the relationships in an alcoholic family, my wife and kids were scared of me, because my behavior was so unpredictable. I was also sleep deprived but felt macho about it, talking myself into believing that I was a tough guy. I mistakenly believed that I was able to withstand sleeplessness while still functioning effectively.

A vacation to Italy gave me a completely new slant on things. That trip was the first step in changing my relationship with food and how that change would also affect my life. We stayed at a boarding school for five weeks, and we ate European style-that meant less beef, lots of vegetables, fewer deep-fried foods. I drank plenty of water and got off soft drinks entirely. And since we had no car, we walked everywhere. I must have taken 10,000 steps a day. I also made it a habit to take a stroll after lunch. With all that walking, my back pain almost went away. Without work, I had no stress, and I found myself sleeping comfortably 8 hours a night. These lifestyle changes came easily and unknowingly, and I lost 20 pounds without even trying!

By the time we got back home, my experience in Europe had convinced me to find a program that concentrated on lifestyle, instead of just dieting. Because I'd heard great things about a program offered by 20/20 LifeStyles, I decided to give it a try.

That first evening, while listening to Dr. Dedomenico's orientation lecture, I had my big "Aha" moment. He was indeed talking about lifestyle and not diets! And he was speaking from the heart, because he was someone who had weighed more than 250 pounds and struggled just like me. He talked about food in ways I could relate to. Yes, I said to myself, this guy knows what I'm going through. Everything he says makes absolute sense.

As I entered into the program, I learned that many of my problems were chemically related. I was diagnosed as insulin resistant and pre-diabetic, which wasn't much of a surprise, since my grandmother had been treated for diabetes. I also came to believe there was something in my genetic make-up that made me prone to weight gain.

With lifestyle counseling, exercise, meal tracking, and the compassion I experienced from the 20/20 LifeStyles staff, I was given the support that enabled me to lose an amazing amount of weight. When I entered the program I weighed 305 pounds-now I'm 197 pounds, and I feel incredible. I'm a lean, mean machine. My fun times involve family, sports, and friends instead of food binges. I'm no longer depressed, and my family likes having me around.

The most important thing I learned was how to establish new habits that would change my daily life.

The fact is, I'm a food addict. And, like an alcoholic, I have to be very careful about falling back into destructive behavior. I have to be vigilant and live my life one day at a time. My body has a chemical imbalance that needs constant care. I'm always aware of it, especially when I choose to put something in my mouth. I also have blood work done every 6 months to make sure I'm staying on track. And I still follow what I learned in the 20/20 LifeStyles program.

This awareness-this self-knowledge and discipline-is the tool I need to live a long and healthy life, and it's something I'm passing on to my children. More than anything else I could provide, it's a lasting gift to them.

Rage felt that his eating was truly out of his control. He felt he was a food addict and was both frightened and puzzled by his addiction to food.

CONCEPT #14
How To Make Yourself An Offer You Can't Refuse

Everybody likes a reward. Behavioral psychologists explain everything we do on the basis of rewards and punishments. But how does this work, when the reward is the punishment? You eat the foods you love, and you feel good, but then you feel terrible. It doesn't seem to make sense, does it? Behavioral psychologists can explain that as well: They call it the power of time proximity.

Rewards and punishments are most powerful when they occur as close in time to the behavior as possible. So, the good feeling you get from eating those foods is far more powerful in influencing your behavior than the misery you feel later. You eat the foods containing sugar, fat, and salt and get a rapid stimulation of your reward (pleasure) center. Tomorrow morning you wake up, look in the mirror, and feel horrible. But remember time proximity. The rapid reward of the food is much more powerful in changing your behavior than the delayed punishment felt the next morning. And since that eating behavior is rewarded, you'll do it again and again.

But where does that good feeling come from? It originates in the reward center[16] in our brain. Foods that trigger the reward center are usually those that contain sugar, fat, and salt. Have you ever seen a person eat just one potato chip?

We like these foods even better if they convey a pleasant sensation in the mouth. Once you start eating those foods, it's very difficult to stop. If you do manage to stop, by force of will, you may continue to crave these foods for days. Why is that?

The answer lies in the chemistry these foods create. Foods high in sugar, fat, and salt trigger the release of specific chemicals in your brain: serotonin, endorphins, and dopamine. Most of us have heard about serotonin, as in Prozac. Serotonin is a feel-good chemical. It gives you a feeling of being happy. If, like Rage, you're depressed about your weight, poor health, poor social life, job, family, etc., you know how to fix that. Just eat something rich in sugar, fat, and salt, and you'll feel better immediately.

What about endorphins? Well, most of us have heard of these neurotransmitters as well. They're also feel-good chemicals, but slightly different from serotonin. They calm and relax us, take away all our little aches and pains. Sounds like we're describing the perfect medicine for almost any problem: Just eat a doughnut, and you'll feel great.

---

16. *For more information on reward-center eating see videos in Appendix J under Nutrition.*

But there's another problem-dopamine. Dopamine has the effect of making you hyper-focus on things. In this case, the things you focus on contain sugar, fat, and salt. And once the dopamine hits your brain, well, I'll bet you can't eat just one. If not being able to eat just one weren't bad enough, because of the chemicals released when we eat these foods, we begin craving them, and that craving may continue after satiety and even after that, when you're stuffed. What's even worse, if you have frequent episodes of reward-center eating, the need for these foods actually intensifies, so that your addiction to them gets stronger.

In our plan, you won't be eating foods that trigger this response, because once it's triggered, it cannot be reliably controlled. As you read further, you'll find many ways to stimulate the feel-good chemicals in your brain through the healthy methods of exercise, visualization, and love-none of which will leave you depressed in the morning.

CONCEPT #15
When Too Much Is Never Enough

There's an old saying about alcoholism: One drink is too many, and 1,000 isn't enough. Unfortunately that's true for some overweight people as well. These people suffer from a malady called binge-eating disorder. About 30 percent of people entering any diet program will have binge-eating disorder. Rage's story is a good example.

Binge eaters rarely have long-term success in any weight-loss program unless their binge-eating disorder is treated successfully. If they're not treated, they can gain their weight back rapidly. Additionally, binge eaters can become extremely obese, often with a BMI(17) greater than 45. Research has disclosed genetic links to binge-eating disorder.

---

17. *Body Mass Index-BMI-is a measure of weight versus height. Normal is 18.5-24.9 for adults. This is only an approximate measure of "normal" and can have significant variations based on muscle mass.*

Initial studies note that binge eating often runs in families, and genetic studies indicate a link between the cortisol-receptor gene and binge-eating disorder. Well, that makes sense.

We've known for some time that individuals who take high doses of such steroids as cortisone consume more calories and gain weight. Cortisol is the body's naturally produced steroid and has much the same effect. You obviously weren't responsible for your genetic makeup, so you didn't cause this problem. But before your disorder can be treated you have to be willing to identify yourself as a binge eater.

ARE YOU A BINGE EATER?			
Rapid eating	Do you eat so fast that there's a lag between your eating and your feelings of fullness or over-fullness?	Yes	No
Eating to discomfort	After a large meal, do you have problems moving, sleeping, or doing your normal routine?	Yes	No
	Do you feel noticeably uncomfortable?	Yes	No
Eating when not hungry	Do you eat even when you've recently eaten or are not hungry?	Yes	No
	Do you find yourself eating again shortly after you've eaten a full meal?	Yes	No
	Do you find yourself going back for seconds or thirds?	Yes	No

Hiding your eating	Do you hide your types and quantities of foods to conceal evidence of your eating from others?	Yes	No
Eating alone	Do you prefer to eat alone so you can eat as much as you want, of what you want, without embarrassment?	Yes	No
Feeling out of control with your eating	Do you feel that you should stop eating but cannot?	Yes	No
	Do you make vows and promises to yourself about your eating and break them quickly?	Yes	No
	Do you make promises to others about your eating, then feel shame when you fail?	Yes	No
Feeling guilt, shame, or disgust about your eating	Do you avoid social eating situations for fear that you might embarrass yourself?	Yes	No
	Do you wake up disgusted with yourself over your eating? Do you feel ashamed of what you ate or how much you ate?	Yes	No
Waking in the middle of the night to eat	Do you eat most of your calories for the day after dinner, or do you wake up and find you're not be able to go back to sleep until you have eaten?	Yes	No

If you answered **Yes** to three or more of these questions, and if you feel this way at least twice a week and it's been going on for at least six months, you may have a binge-eating problem[18].

If you have determined you are a binge eater, then you need to take the following steps to keep that disease from controlling your life, your health, and your lifestyle:

- **Do not hide your food or your eating:** This is a red-flag warning of the return of the disease. You must be totally honest with a support person about your eating. Try to eat with other people and make it a social situation.

- **Do not eat after dinner:** There is a very high rate of association between night-eating syndrome and binge-eating disorder. Be sure to eat meals and snacks during the day so you don't get over-hungry at night.

- **Meal track, meal track, meal track!** Be sure to write down everything that goes into your mouth within 15 minutes of the meal. Doing it at the end of the day or tomorrow or next week does not work for binge eating. Meal tracking is not only the best way to track your eating behavior, it's also the best way to keep it under control and make it manageable.

- **Do not base your feelings of success or failure on the scale:** The scale is a lagging indicator. That means you can be well into your disordered eating before the scale starts to move, and that could be too late. The best indicator of success or failure is your meal tracker. It is "real time" and can alert you to any problems immediately.

18. *For more information on binge eating disorder, see Disordered Eating video under Lifestyle Series in Appendix J.*

- **Regular and consistent exercise helps binge eaters maintain control:** Be very, very serious about this. Get a workout buddy and commit to that person. It's also a good idea to get a backup workout buddy, so when your workout partner is sick, out of town, or unavailable, you are still committed.

- **Accountability is the key:** Accountability gives you the control you need. Be sure you are accountable to someone for your diet and your exercise. Accountability can be to your spouse, your significant other, or a good friend. Make getting a support group or support person a top priority. We find that most people who return to disordered eating have not taken this vital step.

- **Love yourself:** We have to love ourselves for our successes. Love yourself for your successes, and love yourself when you have lapses. You can't get better by hating yourself.

If you desire, you can stay on Stage 2 of the food plan until you have lost all of your weight, then gradually transition carefully through the stages.

Most individuals with binge-eating disorder have done very well on the 20/20 LifeStyles plan. However, if you find that the suggestions above are not working for you, or that attempting to follow the plan makes your binge eating worse, then you'll need additional help. Check back with your physician, or seek out a psychologist or counselor who is very experienced in working with individuals with binge-eating disorder.

They can help you get back in control of your eating and your life. In the Puget Sound area you can contact our Counseling Center at (425) 462-2776, or go to our website: www.proclub.com/Wellness/Counseling

CHAPTER 5

THE CHEMISTRY OF OBESITY

MY MISPLACED PASSION FOR FOOD
Chris, age 38

If you were looking for a poster boy for oblivious weight gain, it would probably be me. I say that because I grew up thinking that I would eat what tasted good and pass on anything that wasn't scrumptious. Since my family was from New Orleans, we had a rather warped view of menu choices in the first place. Until I was well into my 20s, I considered deep-fried foods a primary food group. We deep-fried just about everything including vegetables, so you can imagine how high the cholesterol numbers in my family might have been. My whole family was overweight, and I was a heavy kid as far back as I can remember. As I look back on it, I really didn't feel out of place, because my whole family was just like me. I was simply used to it. I was never very athletic and never aspired to be, so I wasn't terribly disappointed when I wasn't considered for team sports.

My misguided meal habits remained pretty consistent into young adulthood. For one thing, I was one of those people who made food a special event. I gravitated toward taste without regard to calories. I don't believe I had any emotional hang-ups about eating, I just ate what I wanted, and as much as I wanted. I've learned since then that's called reward-center eating. As a result of my mindless eating habits, including overindulgence in beer, by the time I reached my mid-20s, I found myself at 5 feet 9 and weighing 250 pounds.

76

When I met my wife Bridget, we shared the same propensity for rich foods and enjoyed cooking together, which ultimately led to us both gaining weight. No surprise, then, that I soon reached 300 pounds with a cholesterol count just over 240. And that's when I began to be a bit more conscious of my size. I worked at a large software company and had just been informed that we would have to participate in an involuntary exercise program.

The revelation of how obese I was came one night when I was watching "The Simpsons" on TV. I was particularly attuned to the episode in which Homer Simpson wanted to get out of his company's exercise program by reaching the disqualifying weight of 300 pounds; in the cartoon, individuals weighing more than 300 pounds were allowed to stay home and not participate. To my shock, as I watched the show I realized that I had only recently reached that magic number of 300 pounds, and thereby had become a bit of a cartoon myself. It was then that I had a startling insight: At my age, the weight gain would probably be irreversible and likely continue to increase with dire consequences unless I did something. I also admit to some vanity here, since I had a 20-year high-school reunion coming up, and I couldn't face going to see old classmates at my weight.

My wife reminded me that the PRO Sports Club, to which I belonged, had a specialized health and weight-loss plan. Their 20/20 LifeStyles clinic had been very successful in helping people both lose weight and alter the lifestyle habits that caused a variety of ailments.

Furthermore, 20/20 participants seemed to have perfected the means of maintaining their weight loss. That was important to me, as Bridget was now increasingly aware of weight problems because her health had become a major issue. At the age of 34 she was already on medication for diabetes, high blood pressure, and high cholesterol, with high probability she would be on those medicines for the rest of her life.

Both of us badly needed help. And while we were skeptical people by nature, particularly in regard to diets, Bridget and I decided we would give 20/20 LifeStyles a chance. I must confess that I had very strong feelings about rejecting the whole thing and walking away the moment I sensed any hint of falsity or coercion. Of course, I may have been just looking for an excuse to go back to my mindless eating.

Nevertheless, not knowing what to expect, we attended an introductory seminar conducted by Dr. Mark Dedomenico, founder of 20/20 LifeStyles.

What impressed us immediately was the straightforward, no-nonsense way in which the doctor addressed the issues we faced. We could accomplish our goals, he said, if we were ready. Complete commitment was essential to success; there could be no other way.

Bridget and I had been prepared to play hardball and maybe walk out, putting off the decision as long as we could, but after hearing Dr. Dedomenico's very human and very realistic approach to health issues that went far beyond weight loss, we signed up immediately.

Even though we were going through the program together, we decided to do things individually. Each of us had our own personal trainer, our own registered dietitian, and our own lifestyle counselor. Initially, we thought we didn't need the lifestyles counselors because we could support each other. But when the experts at 20/20 informed us that avoiding that portion of the program would dramatically lower the chances of long-term success, we changed our minds.

I learned a great deal about myself in the process. Primarily, I learned that I could succeed if I took Dr. Dedomenico's advice for total commitment and followed the program to the letter. What I didn't do was get impatient or overshoot my goals.

Bridget and I found some great ways of trying new things-like keeping track of meals. I was a software engineer, and she was a CPA. Both highly mathematically inclined, we looked at the calorie-counting responsibilities much like a bookkeeping ledger, like a budget for any business. It became a question of balancing the meal budget in our lives. We also did nothing to sabotage each other by cheating on food rules or skipping workouts or lifestyle counseling sessions.

To us, all that was quite logical and user-friendly, and because we followed the plan to the letter, we succeeded. However, since I had some personal weight goals that extended beyond the duration of the plan, I gave myself a bonus by extending my program.

I lost 125 pounds, dropping from 310 to my current weight of 185. And Bridget, though she didn't need to lose anywhere near as much weight as I did, not only dropped a few dress sizes, she was successful in getting off all of her meds! That's right-no more meds for high blood pressure or high cholesterol or diabetes.

The promise of 20/20 LifeStyles was achievable, just as Dr. Dedomenico had said when he told us it should be our goal to not only lose weight but do so permanently, without drugs, which many people consider unavoidable.

Take it from Bridget and me: Nothing is unavoidable. If you love and respect yourself, you can establish life-changing habits.

Chris had no idea why he ate the foods he ate. He just kept eating those unhealthy foods and gaining weight because he had been eating those foods his whole life.

CONCEPT #16

What Is A Fine-Tuned Body?

The year 1971 saw publication of American psychologist, B. F. Skinner's book, <u>Beyond Freedom and Dignity</u>. Skinner believed that much of what we do in our lives is not by conscious choice, but because elements beyond our awareness constantly direct our behavior.

Nowhere is this truer than in disordered eating. A whole host of processes-behavioral, physical and environmental-can throw your system out of balance. The result of that imbalance is a disconnect between your goals or desires and your eating behaviors. As Chris pointed out, he had no idea why he was destroying his health, his body, and his life with food. We see now that it really wasn't his fault. In terms of nutrition, from a very young age, his body, his education and his environment were completely dysfunctional.

Suppose that when you think of a certain food you say to yourself, "I love that food." You believe your preference for a certain food is a free choice based on taste, but Skinner would disagree. He would say, rightly, that you've been conditioned to "love" that food. He would also suggest that if you'd been brought up in a different family or a different society you might dislike that same food.

Once you start eating certain foods, your body and your mind become conditioned. Your weight-maintenance system is very complicated and very fragile. If that system is off by only 50 calories a day (a little over ½ ounce of bread), you will gain 5 pounds a year, OR 50 pounds in 10 years! So what are the physical reasons behind Chris's love of unhealthy foods?

Many years ago, researchers observed that there were fat mice and thin mice. They were able to determine that the fat mice were greatly deficient in the hormone leptin[19]. And paradoxically, leptin is produced by fat cells. The researchers concluded that leptin was a hunger moderator. When they investigated leptin's role in human beings, however, they discovered the same thing didn't hold true. Further research revealed that some human beings have "leptin resistance," meaning that for some reason their weight-maintenance system isn't using the leptin, and their appetite isn't suppressed.

In rare cases, leptin resistance can be caused by a lack of receptors for the chemical, but more commonly we have taught ourselves to ignore this potent appetite-suppressing hormone. Sustained high concentrations of leptin, due to the presence of a large number of fat cells, can also cause leptin desensitization. When this occurs, it's because an obese person has pushed his or her body past the point where it can self-regulate.

Ghrelin is another factor in weight maintenance. This hunger-stimulating amino acid is produced when the stomach is empty. Eating a meal will suppress production of ghrelin.

We think it's also important for you to know that not getting enough sleep causes decreased levels of leptin and increases levels of ghrelin. Furthermore, a correlational analysis of sleep patterns with obesity over the last 60 years reveals a perfect match. As sleep levels in this country have declined in the last 60 years, overweight and obesity have increased proportionately[20].

19. For more information on how leptin and leptin resistance cause weight gain and metabolic disorder see Appendix C.
20. For more information on sleep and weight loss, see Sleep videos under Lifestyle Series in Appendix J.

What does this have to do with respecting yourself and respecting your body? Your body needs to be treated lovingly. If you push it with lack of sleep, increased stress, and unhealthy diet, it will not function properly. You will have overridden all your body's systems that try to keep you healthy and fit.

CONCEPT #17
There Is A Diabetes Epidemic

Make no mistake about it: Diabetes is a killer. It is a long, slow, painful way to die, and Chris's wife Bridget was rapidly heading down that path. The 2011 statistics from the American Diabetes Association show that there are almost 106 million people with diabetes and pre-diabetes in the United States, and 2 million new cases are diagnosed annually. This is a disaster, and it's getting worse.

Ninety-seven percent of all diabetes is type 2. That means 97 percent of this disease is caused by our own behavior.

Insulin is a hormone the body produces to help carry sugars from your blood into your cells. Type 2 diabetes is caused by insulin resistance. That means your body's insulin receptors are blocked and cannot bond with the insulin. This blockage makes it difficult for your body's cells to absorb sugars, and since your cells live by burning sugar, that's a major problem.

To make matters worse, when your cells are not getting enough sugar, you produce even more insulin, which sends your body a message: "You need more sugar." Then you feel hungry and want to eat more high-carbohydrate foods. And it gets still more serious. Insulin resistance causes your fat cells to open up and store excess fat, instead of converting it to sugar. So, insulin resistance causes you to eat calories you don't need, and then your body readily stores them as fat.

Insulin resistance also prevents the body from metabolizing fats efficiently, leading to high levels of triglycerides and cholesterol in the blood. Furthermore insulin resistance leads to high blood pressure. We call this combination of insulin resistance, high cholesterol, and high blood pressure "metabolic syndrome." And metabolic syndrome is a strong risk factor for heart attack or stroke.

For more than 25 years we have helped patients break their insulin resistance, so that they are no longer dependent on medications. We do this using diet and exercise. Here's how the 20/20 LifeStyles plan can make that work for you:

Exercise enables the glucose (sugar) transporters in your cells to overcome your insulin resistance and function properly. Your body can then move the glucose into the tissue where it is burned as energy. See Appendix C for a full explanation of how just a couple of weeks of exercise can correct insulin resistance.

The fact is, though, that you can never exercise enough to counteract poor nutrition.

Eating two doughnuts adds 500 calories. To burn off two doughnuts, you have to walk 5 miles. It only takes a few minutes to eat two doughnuts. It takes more than two hours to walk 5 miles.

YOU CAN NEVER OVERCOME A BAD DIET WITH EXERCISE!

Following the nutrition and other guidelines described in this book will help many of you defeat your insulin resistance and reduce or eliminate your need for medications. For others, it will keep you from developing catastrophic metabolic syndrome.

CHAPTER 6

THE SELF-SLIMMING MINDSET

LIFE IS A JOURNEY, HEALTH IS A PATHWAY
Angela, age 50

I was frightened because I had lost contact with who I was. I know that statement may sound ridiculous, because I was a prosecuting attorney with a very successful career. On the outside I functioned well, but on the inside I was a complete mess. I felt lost. I no longer knew what I should feel or who I wanted to be.

There was a great deal of stress in my life, both from my career and the terrible loss I'd suffered when my husband passed away. Even though I'd led a successful life to that point, I no longer had the ability to pull myself together. I was struggling and couldn't find a solution.

Now, I can look back at the root causes of my emotional instability, which I hadn't fully recognized. For me, like a great many other people, the roots of my disorientation began in my childhood with my father, an alcoholic, and my mother, a narcissist.

Having an alcoholic parent created a chaotic household. There was no predicting how the day would begin or end. I never knew if things that were planned would actually occur. Worse than that, I never knew which father would come home that day-the fun dad or the angry, raging monster. My mother tried to compensate for my father's mental abuse with her fantasies and plans for me. Since the family was sick on the inside, she wanted me to look perfect on the outside.

Unfortunately, she constantly criticized my weight. Mom was a beautiful woman who maintained herself well, but as she aged she seemed to transfer her expectations onto me.

She was continually trying to manage my weight and even went so far as to make me take amphetamines. It's hard to assess how much amphetamines distort the childhood learning process, but in my case, already growing up in a difficult environment, the amplification of my stress and my emotions was brutal.

Strangely enough, when I look back at pictures of myself as a young child, I see that I was not fat. My mother's focus on me was clearly part of her avoidance of the real issue of my father's alcoholism. Her misplaced focus continued well into my teens.

I had been taught at a young age that women must be very thin to have any worth. I was a victim of the same misconception that leads to misery for so many young girls, who use dangerous fad diets and put their health at risk due to their belief that being thin is the only way to be accepted and loved.

The more my mother tried to control my food, the more I rebelled. The more I rebelled, the more I ate. And my childhood rebellion with food led to the creation of lifelong habits. Food, not alcohol, had become my drug of choice. When I was frustrated, I would isolate myself, read books, and eat. When I was lonely, I would eat. When I was sad, I would eat. When I was tired, I would eat. When I was celebrating, I would eat. Food became my only source of comfort.

These habits followed me into adulthood, and with the passage of time I found myself significantly overweight. I also developed the accompanying chronic ailment of painful arthritis and suffered from lack of sleep. These just gave me more reasons to eat unhealthy foods.

My self-esteem, which had been damaged by my parents in childhood, became even worse as I matured due to my weight gain. My lack of self-respect led to a long and destructive relationship with a man, which created a constant cycle of self-abuse and brought on other self-destructive behaviors, including smoking.

Years later, after my husband passed away, I relocated. In my new town jobs were difficult to find. In unfamiliar surroundings and unemployed, with my husband gone, I felt completely lost and turned even more to food. However, I was taken in by a group of women from a theology school. They became a social haven for me, and before long I decided to join the seminary and become an ordained minister.

Even with my new profession, I reasoned that I would still find some ways to use my law background. But even while I enjoyed my work, I felt unfulfilled. I was still confused. I was suffering from poor health, and I somehow knew that a mind at peace requires a body at peace. After all my searching, the answer came from a most unexpected direction: the 20/20 LifeStyles program.

Having decided that my weight and health problems needed expert help, I had heard about the 20/20 LifeStyles program from a business associate who had done quite well in it.

I attended the introductory seminar and signed up on the spot. I was very impressed with the knowledge of the staff and their down-to-earth, caring attitude.

What I discovered was that the program not only treated my sick body, it healed my mind and soul as well. Not only were the lifestyle counseling sessions I participated in focused on how to lose weight, get healthy, and live better, they also enabled me to find deep emotional meaning and healing.

Doctor Dedomenico and his staff openly expressed the most sincere and genuine caring I could have hoped for.

My dietitian, my exercise physiologist, and my lifestyle counselor formed a community that was absolutely committed to my welfare. Their encouragement was overwhelming. They even had tears in their eyes as they witnessed my growth, my success, and my joy.

I was astounded that through the 20/20 LifeStyles program I could experience my spirituality more deeply than I ever had. You see, I had been wrong about the role of the body and soul most of my life. My Christian orientation had led me to assume that there was a separation of body and soul, with the soul as the focus and the body simply a vessel. I finally made the connection of the body and soul as being one-since both are the creation of God. And once I integrated my own body and soul, I found that I liked my body a great deal more.

The holistic perception that my body, mind, and spirit are integrated allowed me to treat my body with the same respect I gave my spirit, allowing me to maintain a normal weight for some time now. Frankly, I feel fulfilled on all levels. Thank you, 20/20 LifeStyles!

Angela felt lost in a world of negative self-perception. She kept trying to find an answer but could not. The problem for Angela was that she was looking for an answer and did not know the question.

CONCEPT #18
The Self-Slimming Mindset

At a very early age Angela learned how to think fat. Her mother insisted on trying to manage how she ate and how she looked. This caused Angela to have erroneous self-perceptions. She internalized her mother's thinking, so no matter what she thought or what she did, she perceived herself as too heavy and gave up trying to control her food and her weight.

This is a prime example of the self-fulfilling prophecy: What you think is what you are.

If, as you read Angela's story, you empathized with her and you have a similar problem, in order to change, it's necessary for you to reverse this type of thinking.

> *You're probably asking yourself, "How can I start thinking thin?" That's what we call the self-slimming mindset. For you to achieve that mindset, you must first change your attitudes and perceptions.*

The first step is to try to analyze your self-talk. In other words, analyze what you're telling yourself. What you tell yourself is important for your happiness and your health.

In a study published in JAMA, the journal of the American Medical Association, self-perceptions related to negativity and lack of self-esteem were found to account for a higher risk of illness and death.

Here's an example: You have a social function to attend, but your dress clothes no longer fit. So, you decide to go shopping. You're fearful of this experience, because you previously had trouble finding clothes that looked good on you.

You get to the store and try on an outfit, but it turns out to be too small. The clerk brings you the next size up, and that one's too small as well. Finally, you find an outfit that fits, but it's shapeless and bulky.

On the way home, you start talking to yourself, and the self-talk isn't good. You might say such things as this:

I just can't stand myself.

I'm disgusting.

I'm a total failure.

Who would ever want to be around me?

I just can't go to this event.

I just don't want to be seen in public.

I will never maintain a normal weight.

No matter what I do, I always gain weight.

Diets just don't work for me.

I'm hopeless.

The problem with this self-talk is that if you say those things often enough, you'll believe them. And once they become part of your belief system, your behaviors begin to conform to them. These thoughts become almost automatic, and once automatic, they are very difficult to change. Once you've incorporated those negative beliefs, you're no longer able to accept, respect, or love yourself, making positive change almost impossible.

If you're someone who acknowledges negative self-talk as a problem, here's how to change things: Write out a list of your negative self-talk, even if you find it uncomfortable, because it's the only way to understand and change those thoughts.

And when you look at your list, you'll see that these statements are not rational. They fail the "truth test." The truth test focuses on the facts that lie below the frequently exaggerated emotions. To show how this works, let's take a look at one of the examples of negative self-talk above: "I can't stand myself." This statement implies that you not only dislike yourself, you dislike yourself so intensely that you can't live with it.

This statement doesn't pass the truth test, since you've probably lived with that feeling for a long time. Furthermore, there are undoubtedly times when you don't dislike yourself at all, and there have undoubtedly been times in your life when you actually liked yourself. So this statement is obviously false.

The next step is to write down a rational statement, one that will pass the truth test. That statement might be about your humiliating shopping experience. Sure, you're not thrilled with yourself, but let's try to be reasonable. So, by contrast, a possible rational statement might be this: "I feel bad about not being able to successfully manage my weight."

That rational statement works. It passes the truth test, but it's still incomplete. To complete the statement, you'll have to write, "I feel bad about not being able to successfully manage my weight, but considering the faulty education and information I've been given all my life, it's quite understandable."

If you read the original version of the self-talk statement and then the final version, you can't help feeling more positive.

The final step in redirecting your thoughts is to catch yourself any time your self-talk doesn't pass the truth test. Then, reconstruct the thought as illustrated above and say the new version to yourself. You may have to repeat the rational thought to yourself many times.

Remember, those irrational thoughts have become almost automatic. But if you keep repeating those rational thoughts, eventually they will replace the irrational negative thoughts.

CONCEPT #19

Through Visualization You Can See A Better Self

As we explained previously, your mind uses language to shape your beliefs, but it also uses imagery. Angela saw herself as fat because her mother told her she was fat. That's an example of negative visualization. When you're overweight and see yourself in the "mirror" of your mind, what you "see" may magnify the defect. To help our patients reverse that perspective, we use positive visualizations. We use this technique for motivation, as well as to rehearse some event that might be problematic without positive programming.

To try this exercise, take 15 minutes and go to a quiet place: no telephones, dogs barking, or children shouting. Now sit in a comfortable chair and close your eyes. Breathe deeply five times and exhale much more slowly than you inhaled. Now visualize yourself in one month's time. You're just stepping off the scale, ecstatic with your progress. Now see yourself walking into your closet, where you try on your next smaller size, and it fits perfectly! Now, in your mind's eye, you move to the mirror, and when you really examine yourself, you see that your face, belly, and hips are noticeably smaller. Now sense how happy you feel!

Do this each day for 14 days, and your attitude and motivation will soar.

Let's try another situation.

You've now been doing well on this plan for five or six weeks. You're feeling great about your progress, but you've been invited to your mother's house for dinner. You know your mother's habits: If there are eight people invited for dinner, she will cook for 18. Not only that, she has never allowed a vegetable or fruit in her house. She's the grand master of sugar, fat, and salt-the Queen of Carbohydrates.

What's even worse, this is the food you were raised on-your personal soul food. You have about two weeks to prepare, so what should you do?

Go back to your quiet room for 15 minutes a day. Do the same breathing exercise and then visualize yourself driving up to Mom's house. You walk in the front door and smell all the wonderful foods. You see yourself uncovering the dish that you've brought to the dinner, a dish that's healthy and on your plan. As you sit at the table with your healthy food in front of you, you watch the others ignoring the healthy dish you brought and gorging on carbohydrates instead. Now you flash back to that trip to the store, looking for the outfit that was two sizes too small. You look at Mom's carbohydrate-loaded foods again and actually feel a bit ill. On your way home, you feel like you just pitched a no-hitter. You feel great!

The visualization tool is very powerful. Use it to find and become the slim you.

CHAPTER 7

REAPING THE REWARDS

SEPARATING YOUR IDENTITY FROM YOUR WEIGHT
Evan, age 50

I struggled with my weight for most of my adult life. When I wasn't struggling, it was because I was letting myself go, leading to even more pounds.

I'm sure you know the cycle: You work really hard to lose a few pounds with some dieting and exercise, and then, for whatever reason, hit a stumbling block that sinks you.

For me, it was either the stress at work or family holidays that would blow my plans. Work stress would often mean that my work team was forced to grab quick meals at the office, and as part of the relief in the war room, someone would order pizza, with cupcakes and soda drinks as a chaser. On the family side, my grandmother could be deadly. In my family, both my mom and my grandma believed in loading plates with food and reloading as soon as the food disappeared. It was those huge family-driven caloric events that would send me into a tailspin, even if I had made some progress for a few weeks.

One of the benchmarks in my life was a physical fitness test the Army demanded us all to take during my time in the service. Every year, I'd be unable to complete the test and have to retake the sections I failed until I finally passed. Even then, my scores were so dismal that they closed a lot of doors for me. Unfortunately, the better your fitness score, the better will be your chances for entry into certain military schools, and my results were always bad. I was denied advancement. As a soldier, I found it humiliating.

When I got out of the service, my rollercoaster ride with dieting continued. Even though I would take off the pounds, those pounds returned and brought several of their friends along. Over time, those failures piled up. My perception shifted to where I wasn't just the proverbial fat guy any more, I was also the proverbial fat guy who had failed repeatedly at every diet. My surrender to that identity led to a very real acceptance that I was heading for a life of obesity. I simply got used to the idea of having someone hand me dinner through a car window. I went to the hamburger drive-through so often, I should have had my own private lane.

Of course, accepting myself as the fat guy significantly damaged my social life. It drove me to introversion and made me unwilling to take social or professional risks of any kind. My confidence in being attractive to the opposite sex disappeared completely. I grew accustomed to the idea that no one would date a fat guy. Finally, my activities even with friends were severely curtailed, because I usually couldn't keep up with them physically.

So that's how I began to spend more and more time alone at home with my two buddies, Mr. TV and Mr. Fridge. Things had gotten so bad that I was buying slip-on shoes, just so I wouldn't have to bend over to tie them.

But then four things made me turn the corner:

1. I got tired of being sick and tired.

2. I heard some 20/20 LifeStyles success stories.

3. I was witness to Dad's and Mom's failing health.

4. A friend and co-worker, Todd, who was also overweight, died of a heart attack at age 43, leaving an 8-year-old son.

Todd's death and seeing my father's alcohol-driven obesity, which sent him to one doctor appointment after another for a long list of ailments, made me realize I didn't want to suffer a similar fate. In truth, it terrified me.

When I finally looked into 20/20 LifeStyles, I decided to go to the introductory seminar to find out why there had been so many successes. Doctor Dedomenico's two-hour orientation was completely different from what I had expected. Among other things, Dr. Mark spoke about far-reaching holistic avenues to a better life, not just weight loss. I listened carefully, but my aptitude for failure was so deeply ingrained that I couldn't commit. Even so, after I went home, the discussions from the meeting kept echoing in my mind. For the next six months, I began to practice some of those health tips. I cut down on soft drinks dramatically, stopped eating as much fast food, and with some daily exercise, was quite amazed that I actually lost 30 pounds-something that would have been significant, except I needed to lose an additional 70.

I realized I had reached my limits. This was normally the point where I always blew it. I needed the support of the entire 20/20 program, which included a great deal more than my own efforts: lifestyle advice, plus prescribed exercise techniques and dietary regimens so specific that I simply couldn't have come up with them on my own.

As I got into the program, I found the staff so caring and the advice so superior, it immediately put me on the path to success.

The highlight of this experience was the reversal of my previous exercise failures. As I got stronger, my personal trainer wanted to demonstrate my progress by putting me through the same physical fitness test I had always failed in the Army. I was astounded to see the results: In completing the test at the age of 49, I was exceeding the average performance of many 20-30 year olds.

That moment was when I realized that 20/20 LifeStyles had been structured to empower me. The emphasis was always on a positive outcome, and the results were more gratifying than I could have imagined. Overall, I lost the extra weight, for a total loss of 100 pounds.

My ability to exercise and excel became my biggest thrill. Before joining the program, I struggled to climb 14 steps. I was now without limitations. As part of the program they gave me a pedometer and told me I needed to accumulate 5,000 steps a day as a starter. I set benchmarks as I went: 6,500 steps, then 10,000 a day. Believe it or not, on some days, I did 35,000 steps.

What that meant, was a lot of mountain hiking. The farther I climbed, the more that became my new high. I now routinely take 12-14-mile hikes in the Cascade Mountains, on the most rugged terrain I can find. I even have difficulty getting others to hike with me, as most of them find those routes too challenging. The other day I climbed a mountain and set my own record of 52,766 steps-the equivalent of climbing the stairs in a 421-story building.

Am I proud of my fitness? As a previous fat guy who had exercise embarrassment and had been a couch potato, you bet I am. But what I'm proudest of is my story, which I try to share with any and all listeners. I dearly want to help others put their lives back into focus for better health and a longer life.

The other day Dr. Mark told me that I now have a new problem: Since I'm obviously going to live to 100, I should be concerned that I may outlive my retirement funds. My response: Who's thinking about retirement? I've got too many people to help and too many mountains to climb.

It took the premature death of a friend to shock Evan into action. Until that time he was in denial of the fatal nature of his disease.

CONCEPT #20

How Your Waistline Is Damaging Your Health

As Americans have gotten heavier over the last 50 years, another major change has happened. Instead of carrying their weight on their hips and thighs; like Evan, they are now carrying more of this weight on their waist and abdomen. We're finding this in both men and women. Fat around the waist and abdomen is called interior visceral abdominal fat, and it is even more dangerous to your health than other fat deposits.

This visceral fat causes the body to produce more of the chemicals that cause high blood pressure, high cholesterol, diabetes, osteoarthritis, cancer, hardening of the arteries, stroke, and metabolic syndrome. As we've already explained, metabolic syndrome is a leading risk factor in cardiovascular disease.

The production of visceral fat is mainly caused by consumption of grains (especially refined grains), alcohol, and high-fructose corn syrup. A stressful lifestyle and lack of sleep will cause even more fat to be deposited as visceral fat.

Visceral fat also causes and worsens knee and hip problems. Not only does the extra weight cause more wear on the joints, the visceral fat pad also releases chemicals that cause inflammation throughout the body, especially in the hip and knee. In addition, these inflammatory chemicals attack the lining of your blood vessels, making you more likely to have a heart attack or stroke.

If your normal routine, before starting the 20/20 LifeStyles plan, is to get up in the morning and have cereal or some other grain for breakfast, at that moment you've already started an unhealthy cycle.

Your blood-sugar levels quickly rise, and as they do, your insulin level rises with them. The insulin does what it can to help the blood sugar enter your cells, and afterward your blood-sugar level declines, but your insulin level doesn't decline as rapidly. So, about 90 minutes later, you're looking for something to increase your blood-sugar level. You experience that falling blood sugar as hunger, driving you to find more sugars or carbohydrates to eat. As a result, your visceral abdominal fat pad continues to grow, further destroying your health. But here's the good news: The 20/20 LifeStyles plan will reduce that visceral fat to normal levels.

CONCEPT #21
Why Do We Feel Hunger?

Many overweight people have a distorted concept of hunger.

Perhaps you eat for a number of reasons other than true bodily hunger. These reasons can be emotional disturbances, cravings, cueing, seeing others eat, reward-center eating, or habit eating. That's one of the reasons the 20/20 LifeStyles plan emphasizes eating based on time, rather than on what you feel.

In order to control your appetite and not regain your weight, you need to understand how your body works, why you crave certain foods, and how to control your impulses. We've talked about the hormone ghrelin and how its release creates hunger. This hormonal release can increase as you lose weight, making you more aware of being hungry, which is why it's important for you to eat your three meals and snacks on time.

You must also remember to keep an adequate amount of fat in your diet. We believe the minimum is 20 percent. The majority of these fats need to come from such healthy, unsaturated sources as nuts, seeds, avocado, olive oil, etc. So bacon doesn't quite cut it. If you don't have an adequate fat intake, your hunger increases much as it would if you were eating too many simple carbohydrates.

Sugar alcohols can be another cause of hunger, because they add calories without creating satiety. Sugar alcohols occur naturally in plant products such as fruits and berries. They are also often used in foods as sweeteners and bulking agents. Used as a sweetener or sugar substitute, they provide fewer calories than regular sugars. One gram of sugar alcohol delivers, on average, 2.4 calories, as compared to 4 calories from one gram of sugar. Common sugar alcohols are mannitol, sorbitol, xylitol, and isomalt. Because they break down slowly during digestion, these sugar alcohols require little additional insulin to be transported and thus don't cause sudden increases in blood-sugar levels. This makes them popular among diabetics and for use in diet foods.

Some products labeled "sugar free" including hard candies, cookies, chewing gum, soft drinks, and throat lozenges often contain sugar alcohols. You might believe the label "sugar free" means "calorie free," but that's not the case. Sugar alcohols deliver about 30 percent fewer calories than regular sugar. However, in order to create the sweetness of sugar, 30 to 50 percent more of the sugar alcohol is needed, which means there's no calorie saving. Another problem with sugar alcohols is that they speed transit time through the gastrointestinal tract, which often leads to diarrhea. Our advice about sugar alcohols is to limit them carefully.

Lastly, the government has listed glycerin as a carbohydrate, but this substance doesn't affect blood sugar or insulin levels as much as regular sugar. Derived from animal fats and peanut emollients, glycerin is used in many protein bars to give them a soft texture and make them easy to chew. Glycerin yields 4⅓ calories per gram, which is actually slightly more than sugar. It's also half as sweet as sugar and is used to keep protein bars moist and to plasticize such other foods as fudge, gum, and gelatin. Since glycerin increases blood sugar and insulin less than regular sugar does, and it causes no intestinal side effects, we aren't hesitant to recommend its use in products. Just remember, though, glycerin still has 4⅓ calories per gram.

Now you're learning how to control the foods and food additives you consume. But, because everyone's body works differently, you'll have to find what works for you. All sweeteners, even diet sweeteners, can stimulate hunger in most individuals. Eventually you'll know the foods that will allow you to control your metabolism and hunger[21].

21. For more information on sugars and diet, see Carbs and Sugar videos under Nutrition in Appendix J.

CHAPTER 8

NOW, FOR THE NEW LIFESTYLE

YOU ARE WHAT YOU EAT
Kim, age 52

I didn't have the slightest clue what "You are what you eat" really meant until I turned my life around with 20/20 LifeStyles.

It may all go back to the fact that I was very close to my dad, who died when I was 8 years old. Trying to compensate for my lingering grief, my mom was eager to make me happy, so she kept using food as a way to say she loved me and to keep a smile on my face. Whatever the root cause may have been, I grew up in a culture where, whenever I did something good, I was rewarded with food. Naturally, family celebrations were an extension of that concept, and for us, like most other families, feasting on foods high in sugar, fat, and salt, was a tradition that went with all holidays.

I carried that culture into my young adult life, except that I added another dimension to it, using food to make up for things that went badly. Either way, food became a crutch that I abused with complete disregard for what it meant to my body.

Like many other women nearing middle age, I had pushed the envelope of my weight and my health to the breaking point. Then one day I had a revelation. I realized that the task ahead of me-doing something about it-would be almost impossible without outside help. And so I finally got wise and committed to the 20/20 LifeStyles program.

In addition to losing more than 20 pounds, I gained renewed muscle tone and the thrill of being more fit than I had ever been. I also received a solid education about what my body needed to maintain my new peak performance.

Looking back, it seems natural to me now. It seems quite ludicrous that I was not aware of what my unhealthy eating was doing to me, yet I know that millions of you are misinformed, exactly as I was.

You see, my husband and I ate pizza, pasta, loaves of bread every week, cereals, crackers-all kinds of grain-based products without giving it a thought. That's why, when 20/20 LifeStyles removed grains as a principal part of my diet, I was a bit surprised. But after experiencing the changes in how I felt, it made sense. And, by the way, I became living proof that elimination of grain from my diet worked.

Grains can present digestive problems for a lot of people. They can also slow down or stop weight loss-not something you need when you're trying to regulate your food intake and take care of your body by maintaining a healthy weight.

Refined grains-those found in the white flour most people use to bake and cook, plus those contained in many food products on grocery shelves-are essentially empty carbohydrates. When you eat refined flour, it turns into sugar in your body almost instantly. Even if you try to eat only whole-grain foods, they're more calorie-dense, which means it won't take a lot of whole grains to ruin your calorie quota for the day and pack on some extra pounds.

Long story short, what I did as part of the 20/20 LifeStyles program was to eliminate grains for almost two months. You might think that's a challenge, since we're all so accustomed to having breads, cereals, and pasta as part of our meal pattern. But by substituting more vegetables and protein and getting my carbohydrates almost exclusively from fruits instead of calorie-laden grain-filled foods, I really didn't miss them.

Granted, 20/20 LifeStyles allowed me to make a transition to use limited grains later on, and I had the choice whether I wanted to put some grains back into my menu. As it turned out, I learned to plan meals without them. My body feels so much better now that I'm not eating a high-grain diet.

I was fortunate that the 20/20 LifeStyles program taught me why not eating grains is logical and healthy. After that education, I really didn't want grain-based carbohydrates as the main part of my diet ever again. Plus, my husband and the kids have gotten used to eating more fruits, vegetables, and proteins, and we all look forward to finding new ways of preparing salads and vegetables.

I also learned that if you're going to eat whole-grain snacks at all, which you shouldn't often do, you shouldn't eat them alone, but always with proteins.

As you see, things are different in my family since 20/20 LifeStyles. For one thing, having remembered my own youth, I never use foods as a reward for my kids. On our dinner table you will never find a pasta dish, a pizza, or dinner rolls. Sandwiches are now made with lettuce wraps. And I'll tell you, the lessons my children have learned will be their lifestyle lessons too.

That may be the biggest gift that I received from the 20/20 LifeStyles program. My kids have come to understand that our bodies crave good healthy foods. They also appreciate that the way we're eating now is the way human beings were meant to eat. My whole family values the knowledge that the foods you eat are a meaningful foundation for developing self-acceptance, self-respect, and self-love. In other words, "You are what you eat." I love that.

Kim discovered that she felt and functioned much better after removing grains from her diet. Grains can be a problem for some people, but the vast majority of our patients have been able to tolerate a controlled level of grain consumption with success. That's why we designed our plan as a modified elimination diet. We gradually add foods back into your diet, so you can determine whether any specific foods or food groups cause you problems, or cause you to be hungry. Different individuals have different tolerances and sensitivities to grain products. You must carefully find how many grain servings per day you can tolerate without having your hunger return.

Until Kim came into the 20/20 LifeStyles program, she really didn't know that the way she was eating was harming her body. Only after she began to change her lifestyle and her diet did she discover the difference in how she felt.

CONCEPT #22
Why You Have To Leave The Pack.

We human beings are social animals. That's why you feel more comfortable in the company of other human beings and distinctly uncomfortable in isolation. And, because you are a social animal, you tend to follow the rules of the group. From a very young age you've been taught conformity. And, because of that conformity, more than 300,000 Americans die each year from metabolic disorders. If you add to that the number who are disabled or partially disabled, the consequences are staggering.

> *Your group is NOT a safe place to be! If you want to have a full, healthy, and happy life, you must leave the pack.*

The average American consumes 50 to 60 percent of their daily calories in carbohydrates. And, like Kim, if you're reading this book, your diet is probably even higher in carbohydrate content. To make matters worse, a large portion of those carbohydrates comes from foods that contain high-fructose corn syrup. For instance, soda pop syrup contains 55 percent high-fructose corn syrup and 45 percent sugar.

Our hunter-gatherer ancestors consumed the equivalent of 20 teaspoons of sugar a year-quite a difference between that and the 150 pounds each of us consumes in a year now. Much of this added sugar comes from soft drinks or sugar-sweetened beverages.

One 12 ounce can or cup of soda, sports drink, or sweetened tea contains about 8¼ teaspoons of sugar; a 20 ounce cup contains 14 teaspoons of sugar; a 32 ounce cup contains 21 teaspoons of sugar; and a 64 ounce cup contains 44 teaspoons of sugar. Note that in the picture above, one sugar cube equals one teaspoon of sugar.

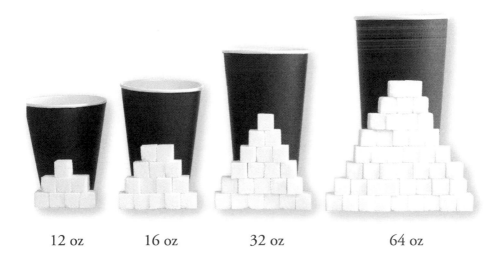

| 12 oz | 16 oz | 32 oz | 64 oz |

High-fructose corn syrup rapidly enters your blood stream and goes directly to your liver, where it causes lipogenesis-production of cholesterol and triglycerides. Furthermore, high intake of high-fructose corn syrup creates a disease called fatty liver. Fatty liver can cause cirrhosis, liver cancer, liver failure, and death.

Make yourself sugar savvy with an awareness of just how much sugar is hidden in your foods. Locate the number of grams of sugar on the label, then divide this number by four to find how many teaspoons of sugar each serving contains. Remember what this sugar is doing to your brain (see Concept #12, Chapter 2).

In this book we will repeatedly refer to product labeling. If you want to understand what you're putting into your body, learning to read product labels is vital. Product labels are not always clear, so we'll try to help you interpret them. Keep in mind that the nutrition label on the package is based on one serving, and many "single-serving" packaged foods are often two or more servings. So you'll need to figure this into your calculations as well.

There are two types of carbohydrates: complex and simple. Simple carbohydrates (simple sugars) are present in such foods as fruit that burn very rapidly in your body. They're great for quick energy but don't provide satiety.

Complex carbohydrates, because of their structure, are high in fiber, so they allow a slower release of sugar into the body. Complex carbohydrates include starchy vegetables, legumes, and whole grains. Complex carbohydrates do not trigger your reward center the way simple carbohydrates do.

Whole grains are complex carbohydrates. This diagram shows you all three components of a whole grain. To truly be a "whole grain" all three components of the grain must be present. The outer bran layer contains the fiber; the inner endosperm is made up of starch (a simple sugar) and antioxidants. The germ contains small amounts of fats and protein.

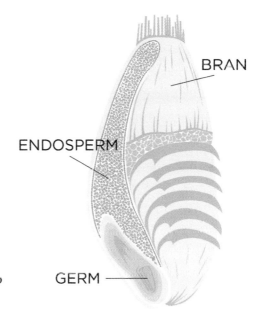

Because bran is very high in fiber, your body has a hard time breaking it down. Hence it releases the starch (sugar) into your bloodstream more slowly, causing a smaller impact on blood-sugar levels.

Some of the grains most commonly consumed are wheat, oats, barley, rye, and brown and wild rice. To make sure something is truly a whole grain, take a look at the ingredient list on the package. For example, if the package states wheat flour as an ingredient, that's deceptive! The ingredient must contain the word "whole" for the item to truly be a whole grain. Be mindful of items like wild rice as well. While these products often say "wild rice" on the package, they're blended with non-whole-grain rice and other carbohydrates. Be diligent when looking for "whole" as the first ingredient in the ingredient label, to make sure your product is truly a whole grain. On wheat breads, look for "100 percent whole wheat" to ensure that the item is a whole grain. Items that say "contains," or "made with whole grain," "high fiber," "12 grain," or "multigrain" are often not whole-grain items. Get comfortable reading the labels on your food, particularly noting the first ingredient on the label, which is always present in the largest amount.

White bread, white rice, and white pasta are examples of refined grains. The grain-refinement process removes all fibrous components of the grain, so both the germ and bran are removed, leaving only the starchy (sugar) endosperm. These food items are cheaper and more stable on the grocery-store shelf. They are also often lower in calories, because removing fiber, protein, and fat removes calories. But don't let this trick you into thinking the refined items are healthier. Remember, starch is metabolized in a manner similar to simple sugars. That's why you may notice that a large plate of white rice or white pasta will not keep you feeling full for long.

Beware! Sugar comes in many forms. Honey actually contains the same basic sugars as table sugar; it just has different proportions of glucose and fructose. So it will set off your reward center the same as table sugar. Other simple carbohydrates or cousins of sugar to avoid include high-fructose corn syrup, agave nectar, molasses, concentrated fruit juices, maple syrup, raw sugar, white sugar, and brown sugar. Remember, when reading labels, any ingredient ending with "ose" is a sugar.

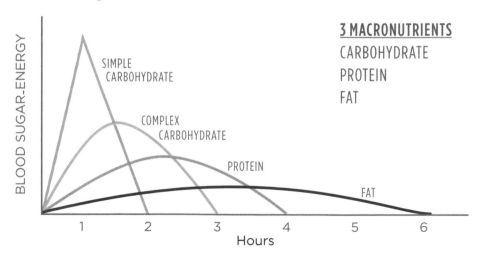

The graph to the left illustrates how the food groups affect your blood-sugar levels over time.

The yellow line demonstrates what happens when you consume simple carbohydrates such as sugar or refined flour. This spike can set off your reward center. The rapid rise, followed by a rapid drop in your blood glucose, stimulates your hunger. The hunger sensation sends you looking for more food, usually something sweet-more simple carbohydrates, sugars, or refined grains. Now look at the blue line. This curve shows what happens when you eat complex carbohydrates, with their slower sugar release. Complex carbohydrates cause no spike and allow a slower blood sugar drop, which doesn't make you hungry. Also, note how the green protein line and the red fat line are fairly flat. These flatter curves represent foods that create satiety, and help stem your hunger for longer periods because your body changes them much more slowly into the sugars it needs. This graph will help you to understand the 20/20 LifeStyles food plan introduced in the next chapter.

In addition to causing you to gain weight and stimulating your reward center, sugar and simple carbohydrates damage your body and brain in many other ways.

A recent study has shown that individuals who consume 10-25 percent of their daily calories in sugars (added to foods) have a 30 percent higher risk of dying from heart disease than those individuals only consuming 8 percent or less of their daily calories in added sugars[22]. This is very disturbing, given all the sugars added to food and beverages by the food industry and by consumers. It's sobering to note that, for daily added sugar consumption, the American Heart Association recommends only 100 calories (6 teaspoons) for women and 150 calories (9 teaspoons) for men. This means that one 12 ounce can of soda, which contains 8¼ teaspoons of sugar, is over the daily limit

22. Q. Yang, et. al., JAMA Intern. Med. February 3, 2014.

for women and almost the entire daily limit for men. So if you consume more than 10 percent of your daily calories in sugar you add to your foods, you are damaging your arteries and your body and your brain. Eating these foods is self-abuse, not self-love.

So, how do you get to be like Kim and break away from the pack? How do you get to break the sugar and carbohydrate habit that's poisoning Americans? Congratulations-by reading this book, you've already started. And, by beginning the meal plan and progressing to Stage 7 of your meal plan, you will have changed your eating habits and your tastes. Your taste buds will become more sensitive, and you'll truly start experiencing the rich flavor and hearty taste of healthy foods.

In order to avoid being drawn back into the pack, you must keep a "top of mind" awareness of what you are doing and why you are doing it. You must remind yourself daily of your reasons for being different.

Make no mistake about it, the pack instinct is powerful. Seeing friends, work associates, strangers, and people on television eating large portions of carbohydrate-laden foods has a powerful effect on you. You want to be part of the group. You want to eat what they eat, and this desire is reinforced by the positive stimulation you get from your reward center when you eat those foods.

Here are a number of ways to help you counter these powerful drives:

- Support of family and friends

- A mentor

- Workout buddies

- Visualizations

- Habit and cue modification

- A picture of yourself at your highest weight on your smart phone, bathroom mirror, laptop, or refrigerator

- Reading sections of this book over again

- Helping others with metabolic problems

- Being involved in a sport or healthy physical activity

The single most important activity you can do to keep this "top of mind" awareness is meal tracking.

Don't stop meal tracking once you've lost all your desired weight, either. You need to continue to meal track at least three days a week for two years after your weight has stabilized.

Time after time, when we've seen patients regain substantial amounts of weight that they had previously lost, they admitted they had not been meal tracking for some time.

CHAPTER 9

LET'S GET INTO ACTION

STAGE 1

No matter what your physical condition may be, it's very important that you check with your doctor before you begin this plan.

The 20/20 LifeStyles nutrition plan has been used to treat many patients with obesity and metabolic disorders, as well as other serious physical ailments.

Almost anyone can engage in this plan, but it's essential to let your doctor see that there is no risk for you personally. It's important for you to do this before you start either the nutrition or exercise portions of the 20/20 LifeStyles plan. It's even more important if you are on medications for diabetes, high cholesterol, high blood pressure, or other disorders. Your doctor may have to adjust these medications when you start the program and as you progress through it.

If you have been given this book by your physician, you know that he/she approves of the 20/20 LifeStyles plan and feels it is safe for you to follow it.

The plan has seven stages with easy-to-follow tips for how to incorporate new foods, with recipes and meal ideas for you to try. Each stage typically lasts one to two weeks or longer, depending on your comfort level and the amount of weight you would like to lose.

You begin with Stage 1, a high-protein meal plan with a controlled quantity of healthy carbohydrates, designed to balance your metabolism and detoxify your body. From there, you add in food groups for each stage and learn how to incorporate these food groups into your meal plan, while assessing your body's reaction to these new foods. Remember, everyone's body is unique, and by adding back foods slowly, you'll be able to identify any reactions or sensitivities you may have to the different foods. These could include hunger, bloating, heartburn, digestive discomfort, skin reactions, or rashes. If you experience any of these reactions you must take that food back out of your plan. In essence, you'll be developing a personal nutrition plan that fits your body chemistry. But remember, unless you meal track in an accurate and timely manner, this technique cannot succeed.

Meal Plan Stages	
STAGE 1: Detox- Lean Protein, Berries, and Healthy Fats	In this stage you will only eat lean protein, berries, and some healthy fats. Berries will provide the carbohydrates you need without causing you to experience hunger or cravings. You will only stay on this stage one week to allow your body to detoxify and your metabolism to become balanced.
STAGE 2: The Basics- Lean Protein, Berries, Healthy Fats, and Vegetables	Stage 2 adds nonstarchy vegetables. With the addition of vegetables, Stage 2 becomes a fully balanced, healthy diet. Many of you may choose to stay on this stage for an extended period of time. Stage 2 is your safe zone, where weight loss is rapid and hunger and cravings are absent.

STAGE 3: Adding Variety- Lean Protein, Berries, Healthy Fats, Vegetables, and High-Protein Yogurt	This stage introduces high-protein (Greek) yogurt. This adds variety to your protein selections, while still keeping you safe from hunger or cravings.
STAGE 4: Apple a Day- Lean Protein, Healthy Fats, Vegetables, High-Protein Yogurt, and Fruit	The introduction of fruit in this stage increases menu options and variety. Fruit is, however, a source of carbohydrates, so portion control becomes very important.
STAGE 5: Dairy Delight- Lean Protein, Healthy Fats, Vegetables, Fruit, and Dairy.	Stage 5 introduces the full dairy selection, including fruit-flavored yogurt, cheese, and milk. This can be a dangerous stage. Some individuals have digestive problems with dairy, some find it causes their hunger or cravings to return, and some find it slows or stops their weight loss.
STAGE 6: Chili Time- Lean Protein, Healthy Fats, Vegetables, Fruit, Dairy, and Legumes.	This stage adds legumes, such as beans, to your plan. Again, this adds variety with foods such as chili or hummus. However, because legumes are high in carbohydrate content, they must be limited.
STAGE 7: The Danger Zone- Lean Protein, Healthy Fats, Vegetables, Fruit, Dairy, Legumes, and Whole Grains.	This is the final stage of the plan. At this point all food groups have been reintroduced into your diet. This is also truly the danger stage. Grains are not a necessary part of your diet, and many of you may have problems with grains. If you find yourself overeating grains or find that grains cause you digestive problems, you will have to minimize or completely eliminate grains from your diet.

In all stages of your plan, meal tracking is absolutely essential. We cannot overstress the importance of tracking, not only during the program, but for at least two years after you reach your goal weight.

Meal tracking ensures that you're meeting your calorie and protein recommendations, but in order to track fully, you must pay close attention to portion size by weighing and measuring your foods. You will notice after tracking religiously for a few months that your knowledge of calories, nutrition information, and portion size will increase dramatically. Nutrition knowledge is a powerful tool, and meal tracking is a great way to learn more about the food you're putting into your body.

Meal tracking also is the best way to determine your body's reactions to the foods you consume because, as we said earlier, everyone's body is different.

Your tracker is the best way to learn about your body chemistry and your sensitivity to various foods.

If you have a slow weight-loss week, the first place to look is your meal tracker. What changed this week? Did you add a new food group? Was your sleep shorter or were your steps fewer compared to previous weeks? Be sure to track your sleep, steps, stress, salt, and hunger in your meal tracker. Then you can use your tracker and really investigate how your body responds, not only to new foods, but also how sleep, stress, and salt affect your hunger, calorie intake, and weight loss.

If your weight loss slows or stops, ALWAYS check the Four Ss: SLEEP, STEPS, STRESS, and SALT.

By now it should be clear that your success on this plan will be directly proportional to the quality of your tracking. Track EVERYTHING you eat, even if you are eating off plan. Do not let guilt sidetrack you into incomplete or inaccurate tracking.

In all stages of your plan, meal tracking is absolutely essential. We promise that, if you meal track properly, within 15 minutes before or after eating, this plan will work for you.

There are many ways to track your food. We recommend our free 20/20 LifeStyles online app as an excellent way to track. You can download your tracker here: www.2020lifestyles.com/get-started/get-started-online/track-it.aspx

On this site you will also find a treasure chest of information related to the 20/20 LifeStyles plan, including more than 60 videos on important health and nutrition topics.

To successfully begin the meal plan, you must first completely clean out your pantry!

Before we get into more detail regarding the Stage 1 meal plan, let's discuss a most important first step to your healthy lifestyle change-cleaning out your pantry!

This includes your pantry, fridge, freezer, office, desk, car, or any other cupboard, nook, or cranny where your junk food and snacks may hide. Yes, all those tempting high-calorie treats must go. Enlist the help of your spouse, family members, or friends in this endeavor. I know you might be saying, "But those pretzels are for the kids!" or "My husband really likes ice cream." Truthfully, your children will learn to follow your lead in healthy eating, and it's essential to have your family completely support you. If they choose to, they can eat their unhealthy foods away from the house.

Having your entire family on board with your
lifestyle change will greatly facilitate your success.

We've included lists of all the foods included on each stage of the meal plan. Let this be your grocery guide each week, as well as a way to keep your pantry full of on-plan foods.

Set a day each week to check your house, and make sure your pantry stays clear of the junk food and snacks. One of the easiest ways to stick to your meal plan is simply to keep off-plan foods out of the house. Your fridge should now be a reflection of your healthy lifestyle. This also means telling your loved ones to avoid bringing home treats or desserts from work or social gatherings. Tell your husband or wife to enjoy those foods at work, but please don't bring them home. If the family wants ice cream, let them leave the house and eat it elsewhere. That way your family can enjoy occasional treats but still support you with a fridge and pantry full of healthy foods.

Changing your eating, your time management, and your lifestyle will be challenging, so you'll need to keep your eye on the target and persevere if it becomes difficult or confusing. In each phase of the plan you'll have numerous food choices, which should enable you to create a menu you enjoy. Appendix J has many tips for preparing healthy ethnic foods, and Appendixes E and G include tasty ways to prepare vegetables and recipes for each stage.

Remember, if you haven't read Chapters 1 through 8, you will not have long-term success with your weight and health. This will just be another diet.

Now you're ready to successfully begin Stage 1.

Stage 1 is the first of seven stages on your journey back to health. We lovingly refer to the first stage of the 20/20 LifeStyles meal plan as our "detox" week. Don't worry, we promise it won't be as difficult as you think. This initial stage is meant to reset your system so that you're no longer battling cravings or hunger. The average American diet, which is heavy in sugar and refined carbohydrates, can lead to spikes and valleys in your blood sugar. Sugar and refined carbohydrates are also responsible for both the production and storage of fat and are the cause of fatigue, irritability, and hunger cravings. The purpose of Stage 1 is to correct these imbalances. Controlling blood sugar is a key to your success in healthy weight loss and a self-slimming mindset. After all, we all make better decisions when we feel our best.

Stage 1 is centered on lean and very lean protein, berries, and healthy fats. This means that, for now, we have taken all grains, and starches out of your diet. Although it looks restrictive, these three components will meet your body's nutritional and satiety needs for this first week. These dietary staples will help your body detoxify. Say goodbye to the sweets, treats, and greasy meats, because after a few weeks you won't even want them anymore. You will also experience a jump-start on your weight loss during this first week, as your body detoxifies and regains its chemical balance.

While you're focusing on weight loss, your calorie goal is 1,100-1,400 calories for women and 1,300-1,700 calories for men. Less doesn't mean better, so make sure to consume at least 1,100 for women or 1,300 for men to get maximum weight loss. Make sure to eat at regular intervals and avoid skipping meals or snacks. None of us makes good food choices when we're hungry, so make sure you have a meal or snack every three to four hours.

Let's discuss the difference between "very lean" and "lean" protein. The proteins listed later in this chapter under "protein options" as "very lean proteins" have too little fat to meet your body's needs. With very lean proteins, you must add a healthy fat serving (see "healthy fat options" later in this chapter). That's right, your body needs fat, but the right kinds and in the appropriate quantities. The proteins listed in the "lean protein" category have adequate fat content, so with those proteins there's no need for extra fat. If your favorite protein is not on the list, avoid it during the early stages of our plan (and this means you, bacon).

Along with protein, healthy fat is crucial for satiety. For your fat servings, we'll be adding one healthy fat serving to your very lean proteins at breakfast, lunch, and dinner. Focusing on unsaturated or "healthy" fats will not only help keep you satiated, it can also help correct imbalances in your cholesterol and triglycerides. Refer to the Stage 1 shopping list later in this chapter for specific fat servings to include, a list of which protein options will need added fat, and which items will not.

Processed meats should only be used sparingly because of their high sodium (salt) content. If you have high blood pressure, avoid them completely. Processed meats include deli meats (such as packaged sliced turkey or ham and all sliced meats from the deli case), precooked packaged meats (such as refrigerated chicken or steak strips), and most frozen proteins (such as breakfast sausage, turkey or salmon burgers, precooked meatballs, etc.). *If you're using a processed meat or fish, aim for less than 500 mg of sodium per serving and only use that food for ONE meal per day.* Limiting processed meats to one meal per day will help you keep your sodium in your target range of 1,500-2,300 mg per day. But be cautious of serving sizes here. If one serving is only 2 ounces and 450 mg sodium, and you need 4 ounces for your meal, that would give you 900 mg of sodium, so this processed meat will not fit into your meal plan.

To avoid relying on processed meats as your sole protein source, consider batch cooking your proteins. For example, make time one or two nights a week to grill enough chicken breasts or lean steaks to last you through the week. This will save you time with meal preparation and planning.

For the first stages of the meal plan, our main source of carbohydrate will be berries. We include berries in Stage 1 to provide energy to your body and fuel for your brain. *Think of berries as their own food group.* They're lower in carbohydrates than the rest of the fruits, and the 1 cup serving will not cause hunger and blood sugar imbalances. The 1 cup serving *only* applies to berries, so we want you to understand that berries are a unique food group; consider them a "safe" carbohydrate. Our bodies need carbohydrates, but we need significantly less than the average American consumes. When you follow your meal plan, know that the allotted servings of berries will be enough carbohydrate to energize you through the day without causing hunger or cravings.

Remember, berries are their own food group. You can have only one cup per meal.

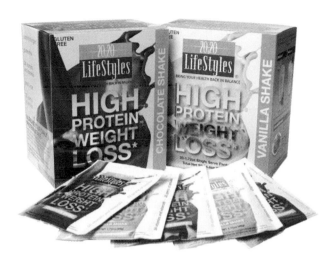

You will notice that we use **20/20 LifeStyles High Protein Dry Powder Shakes**, 20/20 LifeStyles Ready-To-Drink shakes, and 20/20 LifeStyles Protein Bars for convenient options in your meal plans. These are not a required part of your meal plan, and you do not need them to be successful with this plan. You may substitute whole food options for your meals and snacks instead.

Directions on how to prepare the 20/20 LifeStyles High Protein Dry Powder Shakes are located on the back of the package. The 20/20 LifeStyles protein shakes are available in chocolate, vanilla, and strawberry; they provide a high-quality protein source with carbohydrates that will give you energy. Many of our clients use them because they are a great option for a quick, balanced, and satiating breakfast that takes very little prep time.

Eating breakfast is essential to your meal plan because it increases your cell metabolism and helps you burn more calories.

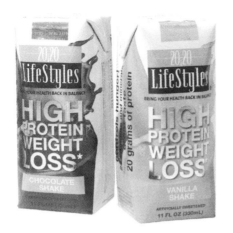

20/20 LifeStyles Ready-To Drink-Shakes are a convenient, high-protein, and shelf-stable alternative to our dry powder shakes. These shakes, available in both chocolate and vanilla, can be used along with 1 cup of berries as a snack option that you can have on the go, without needing refrigeration or a blender. Directions on how to incorporate these ready-to-drink shakes as a breakfast alternative can be found in Breakfast Shake Alternatives later in this section.

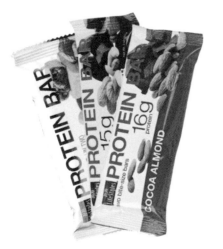

20/20 LifeStyles Protein Bars come in cocoa almond, chocolate peanut, and yogurt peanut crunch. They contain a balance of high-quality protein, carbohydrate, and healthy fat to give you energy and satiety.

Many similar products are on the market, but the ones mentioned here are specifically designed for the 20/20 LifeStyles food plan. The powdered shakes contain 23 grams of whey protein, and the ready-to-drink shakes contain 20 grams of protein. The protein bars are made with inulin, a high-quality prebiotic that helps grow healthy gut bacteria to reduce cholesterol levels.

Caution: If you have dairy intolerance (digestive problems from eating dairy) do not use the dry or the liquid shakes, which contain a dairy protein.

You can find more information on 20/20 LifeStyles High Protein Dry Powder Shakes, ready to drink shakes, and snack bars online: https://shop.2020lifestyles.com/

You may be concerned or anxious about Stage 1, but just know that a great many of our patients come back the second week saying it was much easier than expected. That's because the meal plan is easy to follow; it offers you structure and demystifies the complexity of what normally constitutes a balanced meal.

During Stage 1, include proteins that you enjoy in your meal plan, and find creative ways to prepare them. Don't hesitate to add your favorite herbs and spices to boost the flavor in your recipes. If your chef skills are a bit rusty, now is a great time to polish them up. Take a look at the recipes featured in Appendix H, or view our Stage 1 cooking video online: www.2020lifestyles.com/resources-tools/educational-videos.aspx

We must warn you, the first three days on this meal plan are typically the most difficult. It's not uncommon to experience mild headaches, fatigue, and mild hunger during this time as your body adjusts to the new diet. But not to worry; keep in mind that this occurs because your body is detoxifying from refined carbohydrates. If you experience these symptoms, make sure to eat every 3 or 4 hours, and remember to eat your berries. They're your main source of carbohydrate in the first week, so they're very important. Once you're over the first few days you'll feel much better and not experience hunger. In fact, you might even feel that this meal plan provides you with too much food, but even so, don't skip meals or snacks.

Last, let's quickly discuss water. Water intake is crucial for regulating body temperature, nutrient transport, and rebalancing the good bacteria in your intestinal tract. It's also crucial for satiety. Aim for 64 ounces of water per day-that's eight 8 ounce servings. Use this first week to really make water intake a priority. A slice of lemon or lime can add some flavor to your water, but know that water intake is just as important as following your meal plan. For more information on the importance of water, see Appendix G.

Calorie-containing beverages such as juices, soda, and soup should be avoided, as they do not contribute to satiety. Only calorie-containing beverages with at least 20 grams of protein can be consumed as part of this plan.

Our biggest tip is to embrace this meal plan completely. You'll be thankful you did after you see the first week's promising weight-loss results. Stage 1 lasts for one week. Congratulations on taking your first step to a happier and healthier you!

Now for the specifics.

MEAL PLAN: DETOX

This stage includes: Very lean and lean protein, berries, and healthy fats

Serving Sizes: The ounce measurements for protein refer to cooked weight. Weigh your protein after it is cooked. You will need to measure your berries, and the cup needs to be level, not heaping.

Women

4 ounces protein for breakfast

4 ounces protein for lunch and dinner

1 cup per meal and snack.

Men

4 ounces protein for breakfast

6 ounces protein for lunch and dinner

1 cup per meal and snack.

Healthy fat options (add to very lean protein only):

One fat serving = 45 calories, 5 grams fat. Here's a list of ideas:

- 1 teaspoon oil

- 6 almonds

- 10 peanuts

- ⅛ avocado

- 10 black olives

- 1 tablespoon seeds (sesame, sunflower, pumpkin)

- 1 tablespoon low-fat mayonnaise

- 2 tablespoons low-fat salad dressing

- 1 teaspoon butter or trans-fat-free margarine

- 1 tablespoon natural peanut or nut butter (Natural nut butters should have no added sugar or oil on the ingredients label.)

SHOPPING LIST

- ☐ Food scale (preferably electronic)

- ☐ Measuring cups and spoons

- ☐ Berries - Fresh or frozen (no syrup added; unsweetened if using frozen): blueberries, blackberries, raspberries, strawberries. Cranberries are NOT included because of their high sugar content.

- ☐ Optional items: 20/20 LifeStyles High Protein Dry Powder Shakes, 20/20 LifeStyles Ready-To-Drink Shakes, 20/20 LifeStyles Protein Bars. Available at: https://shop.2020lifestyles.com/

Protein options:

Very lean proteins: Chicken breast (skinless), turkey breast (skinless), low-sodium deli chicken or turkey. Canned tuna (limit to 2 servings per week), fresh or frozen tilapia, cod, halibut, or shrimp. Ground beef (no more than 4-5 percent fat). Venison, bison. Liquid egg whites, Egg Beaters, or other egg substitutes.

Lean proteins: Salmon, pork tenderloin, lean beef (sirloin steak, filet mignon, flank steak, tenderloin, and rib, chuck, or rump roast), low-sodium deli ham. Ground beef (10 percent fat). Dark-meat poultry without skin.

Healthy fats: Olive or canola oil or spray, natural peanut butter, low-fat mayo, almonds, avocado.

Spices/flavorings: Lemons/limes, garlic, ginger, green onions, parsley, red pepper flakes, basil, oregano, mustard, cumin, paprika, vinegar, etc.

Note: Limit those options that contain sugar or salt as an ingredient.

Beverage options: Mineral water, Talking Rain with fruit essence (without sweetener), herbal teas, decaf coffee, green or white tea.

Note: These beverages are not required on your meal plan.

Limited beverages: Coffee, no more than 8 ounces black drip coffee or 2 shots espresso per day. Regular tea, no more than 16 ounces per day.

Supplements: A good one-a-day multi-vitamin [23].

Vegetarian Proteins: If you do not eat meat, poultry, or fish, you must follow the following guidelines:

To ensure adequate protein intake with vegetarian protein options, make sure you read the label.

1 ounce of protein = 7 grams. For women, make sure you consume 28 grams of protein per meal. Men need to consume 42 grams.

Vegetarian very lean proteins

- High-protein tofu: Azumaya Lite, Sol Cuisine.

- TVP (textured vegetable protein).

Vegetarian lean protein options

- Soy products (hamburger-style soy burgers or patties, deli meat, meat balls, hot dogs). Brands like BOCA, Morningstar Farms, Beyond Meat. Avoid garden-burger style, as they may contain grains.

23. For an explanation of what supplements you should take and why you should take them, see Appendix N.

- High-protein tofu. Brands: Wildwood.

- Other options: Nutrela, Tempeh.

Nonfood items you will need: A good pair of running shoes as described later in this chapter under Stage 1 Exercise. A heart-rate monitor, described in the same section. A good 3 axis pedometer like Fitbit or Microsoft Band.

STAGE 1

Women 1,100-1,400 calories

BREAKFAST	CALORIES	FAT (g)
4 ounces very lean protein	140	0-4
2 heart-healthy fat servings *(see list for options)*	90	10
1 cup berries	80	0

Breakfast Alternatives

If you would like to replace your protein, berries, and two healthy fat servings at breakfast for a high-protein shake, follow these guidelines for a quick, tasty, balanced alternative.

High Protein Dry Powder Breakfast Shake Blend:
- 1 packet 20/20 LifeStyles High Protein Dry Powder
- 1 cup water
- 5-6 ice cubes
- 1 cup berries
- 1 tablespoon natural peanut butter or nut butter

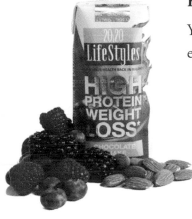

High Protein Ready-To-Drink Breakfast Shake

You may blend these 3 ingredients together or eat/drink them separately.

- 1 20/20 LifeStyles High Protein Ready-To-Drink shake
- 1 cup berries
- 1 tablespoon natural nut butter OR 6 almonds OR 10 peanuts

LUNCH	CALORIES	FAT (g)
4 ounces very lean/lean protein	140-220	0-12
1 heart-healthy fat servings *(add to very lean protein only)*	45	5
1 cup berries	80	0

SNACK *(1 per day between lunch and dinner)*	CALORIES	FAT (g)
Choose ONE of these options for your snack:		
2 ounces very lean protein	130	0-2
20/20 LifeStyles High Protein Dry Powder Shake plus 1 cup berries *(NO peanut butter)*	260	0
20/20 LifeStyles Ready-To-Drink Protein Shake plus 1 cup berries *(NO peanut butter)*	220	6

20/20 LifeStyles Protein Bars - On the Go Snack Option

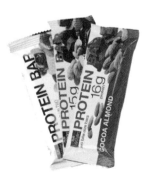

The 20/20 LifeStyles Protein Bars are not a required part of this meal plan. But for times when you are on the go and need a high-protein, shelf-stable snack, they are very handy. The 20/20 LifeStyles Protein Bars are available in chocolate peanut, yogurt peanut crunch, and cocoa almond flavors. Use them as a replacement for your snack when you need a quick one.

Only consume ONE protein bar per day to keep your daily calories and fat in range.

DINNER	CALORIES	FAT (g)
4 ounces very lean/lean protein	140-220	0-12
1 heart-healthy fat servings *(add to very lean protein only)*	45	5
20/20 LifeStyles High Protein Dry Powder Shake plus 1 cup berries *(NO peanut butter)*	260	0

Healthy fat options *(add to very lean protein only):*

> One fat serving = 45 calories, 5 grams fat. Here's a list of ideas:
> - 1 teaspoon oil
> - 6 almonds
> - 10 peanuts
> - ⅛ avocado
> - 10 black olives
> - 1 tablespoon seeds (sesame, sunflower, pumpkin)
> - 1 tablespoon low-fat mayonnaise
> - 2 tablespoon low-fat salad dressing
> - 1 teaspoon butter or trans-fat-free margarine
> - 1 tablespoon natural peanut or nut butter*
> *Natural nut butters should have no added sugar or oil on the ingredients label.*

SAMPLE MENU

DAY 1

BREAKFAST:

- 20/20 LifeStyles High Protein Dry Powder Shake

- 1 tablespoon peanut butter

- 1 cup blueberries

LUNCH:

- 4 ounces baked salmon with a splash of lemon juice and 1 teaspoon chopped dill

- 1 cup strawberries

SNACK:

- 20/20 LifeStyles Protein Bar

DINNER:

- 4 ounces chicken breast

- 1 teaspoon oil for cooking

- 20/20 LifeStyles High Protein Dry Powder Shake plus 1 cup berries *(NO peanut butter)*

DAY 2

BREAKFAST:

- Scramble 8 egg whites, using 1 teaspoon olive oil

- Dash paprika for flavor if desired

- 1 tablespoon nut butter

- 1 cup strawberries

LUNCH:

- 4 ounces canned tuna mixed with 1 tablespoon reduced-fat mayo and avocado

- 1 cup mixed berries

SNACK:

- 2 ounces chicken breast without skin

- 1 cup blueberries

DINNER:

- 4 ounces filet mignon with dash of pepper

- 20/20 LifeStyles High Protein Dry Powder Shake plus 1 cup berries *(NO peanut butter)*

DAY 3

BREAKFAST:

- 4 ounces turkey breast

- ¼ avocado

- 1 cup blackberries

LUNCH:

- 4 ounces very lean ground beef (4-5 percent fat) cooked with Italian seasoning and chopped garlic

- 6 almonds

- 1 cup strawberries

SNACK:

- 2 hardboiled eggs*

- 1 cup raspberries

* If hardboiled eggs are used for a snack, limit consumption of eggs to 2 whole eggs daily.

DINNER:

- 4 ounces grilled salmon with splash of fresh lemon

- 20/20 LifeStyles High Protein Dry Powder Shake plus 1 cup berries (NO peanut butter)

STAGE 1

Men 1,300-1,700 calories

BREAKFAST	CALORIES	FAT (g)
4 ounces very lean protein	140	0-4
2 heart-healthy fat servings *(see list for options)*	90	10
1 cup berries	80	0

Breakfast Alternatives

If you would like to replace your protein, berries, and two healthy fat servings at breakfast for a high-protein shake, follow these guidelines for a quick, tasty, balanced alternative.

High Protein Dry Powder Breakfast Shake Blend:
- 1 packet 20/20 LifeStyles High Protein Dry Powder Shake
  1 cup water
- 5-6 ice cubes
- 1 cup berries
- 1 tablespoon natural peanut butter or nut butter

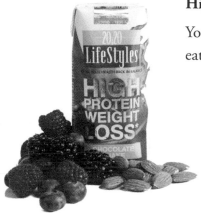

High Protein Ready-To-Drink Breakfast Shake

You may blend these 3 ingredients together or eat/drink them separately.

- 1 20/20 LifeStyles High Protein Ready-To-Drink Shake
- 1 cup berries
- 1 tablespoon natural nut butter OR 6 almonds OR 10 peanuts

135

LUNCH	CALORIES	FAT (g)
6 ounces very lean/lean protein	210-330	0-18
1 heart-healthy fat servings *(add to very lean protein only)*	45	5
1 cup berries	80	0

SNACK *(2 per day; one between breakfast and lunch and one between lunch and dinner)*	CALORIES	FAT (g)
Choose ONE of these options for your snack:		
2 ounces very lean protein plus 1 cup berries	130	0-2
20/20 LifeStyles High Protein Dry Powder Shake plus 1 cup berries *(NO peanut butter)*	260	0
20/20 LifeStyles Ready-To-Drink Protein Shake plus 1 cup berries *(NO peanut butter)*	220	6

20/20 LifeStyles Protein Bars - On the Go Snack Option

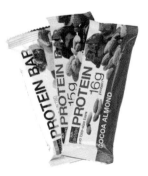

The 20/20 LifeStyles Protein Bars are not a required part of this meal plan. But for times when you are on the go and need a high-protein, shelf-stable snack, they are very handy. The 20/20 LifeStyles Protein Bars are available in chocolate peanut, yogurt peanut crunch, and cocoa almond flavors. Use them as a replacement for your snack when you need a quick one.

Only consume ONE protein bar per day to keep your daily calories and fat in range.

DINNER	CALORIES	FAT (g)
6 ounces very lean/lean protein	210-330	0-18
1 heart-healthy fat servings *(add to very lean protein only)*	45	5
20/20 LifeStyles High Protein Dry Powder Shake plus 1 cup berries *(NO peanut butter)*	260	0

Healthy fat options (add to very lean protein only)

One fat serving = 45 calories, 5 grams fat. Here's a list of ideas:

- 1 teaspoon oil

- 6 almonds *(unsalted)*

- 10 peanuts *(unsalted)*

- ⅛ avocado

- 10 black olives

- 1 tablespoon seeds *(sesame, sunflower, pumpkin)*

- 1 tablespoon low-fat mayonnaise

- 2 tablespoon low-fat salad dressing

- 1 teaspoon butter or trans-fat-free margarine

- 1 tablespoon natural peanut or nut butter*

* *Natural nut butters should have no added sugar or oil on the ingredient label.*

SAMPLE MENU

DAY 1

BREAKFAST:

- 20/20 LifeStyles High Protein Dry Powder Shake

- 1 tablespoon peanut butter

- 1 cup strawberries

SNACK:

- 2 ounces grilled chicken

- 1 cup blackberries

LUNCH:

- 6 ounces salmon with dash of lemon juice plus 1 teaspoon chopped dill

- 1 cup strawberries

SNACK:

- 20/20 LifeStyles Protein Bar

DINNER:

- 6 ounces chicken breast grilled with 1 teaspoon olive oil

- 20/20 LifeStyles High Protein Dry Powder Shake plus 1 cup berries *(NO peanut butter)*

DAY 2

BREAKFAST:

- Scramble 1 cup Egg Beaters, using 1 teaspoon olive oil

- Dash paprika if desired

- 1 tablespoon nut butter

- 1 cup strawberries

SNACK:

- 2 ounces low-sodium deli turkey

- 1 cup raspberries

LUNCH:

- 6 ounces canned tuna mixed with 1 tablespoon reduced-fat mayo

- 1 cup mixed berries

SNACK:

- 2 ounces chicken breast, such as rotisserie without the skin

- 1 cup blueberries

DINNER:

- 6 ounces filet mignon

- 20/20 LifeStyles High Protein Dry Powder Shake plus 1 cup
  berries *(NO peanut butter)*

DAY 3

BREAKFAST:

- 20/20 LifeStyles High Protein Dry Powder Shake

- 1 cup blueberries

- 1 tablespoon peanut butter

- 1 tablespoon unsweetened cocoa powder for flavor

SNACK:

- 2 ounces grilled chicken breast

- 1 cup blackberries

LUNCH:

- 6 ounces very lean ground beef, cooked with Italian seasoning and chopped garlic

- 6 almonds

- 1 cup strawberries

SNACK:

- 2 hardboiled eggs

- 1 cup raspberries

DINNER:

- 6 ounces grilled chicken breast

- 5 walnut halves

- 20/20 LifeStyles High Protein Dry Powder Shake plus 1 cup berries *(NO peanut butter)*

SUMMARY FOR NUTRITION

This week, let's make it simple. We want you to make seven nutritional lifestyle changes.

1. Consistently track your meals and snacks on your 20/20 LifeStyles app or any meal tracker you prefer.

2. Make sure to eat at least 1,100 calories for women, 1,300 calories for men.

3. Eat three meals and one snack for women, two snacks for men. No deviation.

4. Eliminate all sodas and diet sodas from your diet.

5. Limit yourself to 1 cup regular coffee per day. We do not recommend using artificial sweeteners, but if you need one, use Stevia, sparingly.

6. Consume 64 ounces of water daily.

7. Take a daily multivitamin designed for men or women. Also, be sure to see Appendix N for your supplement needs. You can find these supplements online: www.2020lifestyles.com/

As you read through the sample menus in these chapters you will see instances where 20/20 LifeStyles shakes and bars are used in a meal or snack. You can substitute 2 ounces very lean protein for a ready-to-drink shake and 2 ounces of very lean protein plus a serving of berries for a bar or a dry powder shake. See Appendix M for more options.

EXERCISE PLAN: START MOVING

We'd like to remind you again: At the beginning of this chapter we explained why it was important to talk to your doctor before you start this program and to make sure your doctor monitors your progress, if necessary. Be sure to follow this recommendation! Additionally, if you're having problems with the exercises, you can contact a personal trainer to suggest alternative exercises for you. Or, if you live in the Puget Sound area, you can make an appointment to see one of our exercise physiologists by calling (425) 861-6258 or (877) 559-2020, or by email to 2020lifestyles@proclub.com.

As readers of this book may have great variability as to their readiness for exercise and level of fitness, we will break down exercise recommendations into three fitness categories.

We recommend a minimum of five days per week for exercise, but you should note that exercising six days will increase the speed of your weight loss [24].

Level 1: Low fitness or deconditioned- These individuals have sedentary jobs and lifestyles. They get winded just walking up two flights of stairs. They have not participated in formal exercise or sports in at least a year.

Level 2: Moderate fitness or fairly active- These individuals have active jobs and/or lifestyles. They're physically active at least 20 hours per week. They may work physically demanding jobs that require lifting heavy objects or walking long distances. They may work out moderately two to three times per week. They may be involved in a moderately active sport such as skiing, snowboarding, or baseball.

Level 3: High fitness or very active- These individuals are very physically active. They participate in very vigorous activity at least three days per week. This activity could be running for 45 minutes, working at least 20

24. *See video on Exercising and Having Fun under Exercise in Appendix J.*

hours per week at a strenuous labor-intensive job, or playing a very active sport, such as soccer, two to three days per week.

EXERCISE

Level 1: Low fitness- Moderate-speed walking for 20 minutes at least five days per week. Moderate means breathing hard, but having enough breath to speak in full sentences. This will require a good pair of running shoes. Do not try to save money on running shoes; the price you pay will be foot and joint pain and inability to complete the plan. A good pair of shoes will cost about $100. Your local sports store can recommend the best pair for your foot, weight, and usage. If you have foot problems, you must resolve those before you start the exercise program. See your doctor, a podiatrist, or, if you live in the Puget Sound area, schedule an appointment with our podiatry department at (425) 861-6254.

Level 2: Moderate fitness- High-speed walking for 30 minutes at least five days per week. You should keep your heart rate near mid-range level as described below. This will also require a good pair of running shoes, as well as a heart-rate monitor. Several good heart-rate monitors may be purchased at most sports stores or at https://shop.2020lifestyles.com/c-9-gear-accessories.aspx. Find one that is comfortable for you to wear while exercising.

Here is how you figure your optimum heart rate: Take 220 and subtract your age, then multiply by 65. This equals the low end of your optimum heart rate. Next, take 220 minus your age, then multiply by 85. This equals the high end of your optimum heart rate.

Let's look at an example. If you're a 40-year-old person, your age-predicted heart rate would be 220 minus 40 = 180. Now 180 times 65 = 117. Next, we take 180 times 85 = 153. So, when exercising, you would want to maintain your heart rate to be between 117 and 153. Pretty simple.

Level 3: High fitness- Running 30 minutes for at least five days per week. Heart rate at optimum level. Same equipment as moderate level. If you are already doing more than this, continue to do it.

Follow the exercise guidelines in this book and do not overexercise. If you do, you will cause your body to go into starvation mode and slow your weight loss. You can also cause injury, which will delay your program.

LIFESTYLE PLAN: START CHANGING

The goal for your exercise in Stage 1 is simply to get moving. Stick with this simple exercise routine to avoid doing too much, too soon. Remember, we want this lifestyle to last. Performing your exercise in this manner will help prepare your body for the physical challenges to come.

There is a pervasive myth that the less you sleep, the more calories you burn, so sleeping less should be slimming. WRONG! Your body produces a number of chemicals during deep sleep that actually curb appetite. Additionally, if you are sleep-deprived, you have a marked reduction in NEAT[25]-non-exercise activity thermogenesis. Thermogenesis is defined as heat production, and because heat is measured in calories, thermogenesis is how we burn calories. Many things we do during the day create NEAT. People who fidget create more NEAT than people who sit quietly. People who slouch create less NEAT than people who sit up straight. People who gesture actively with their hands create more NEAT.

In some revolutionary research on NEAT at the Mayo Clinic, Dr. James Levine showed that the difference in NEAT between individuals

25. See video on Metabolism and NEAT under Lifestyle Series in Appendix J.

can be as much as 3,500 calories per day! Yes, 3,500. That's roughly equal to one pound a day of weight loss. So, reducing the amount of NEAT you produce if you're sleep- deprived is not a small matter. You need a minimum of 7 hours sleep per night. If you can't do that, you will be continually pushing a rock uphill in your attempts to maintain a healthy body weight. If you have difficulty sleeping, talk to your doctor about it. It's important.

Hard to find the time to sleep and the time to exercise? Well, let's talk briefly about time management. No exercise, no sleep, and fast foods are ways that some of us choose to save time. The problem with this approach is that by taking these shortcuts you're destroying yourself. Statistically, you won't save time. In fact, you'll lose time, because you will die many years before you would if you were healthy. Start planning what you intend to give up or how you will modify your schedule to get the time to lead a healthy life. Remember, time is not elastic; it doesn't stretch, so to put something in, you must take something out. We'll talk a lot more about time management in Chapter 11.

Now some of you may be thinking, "That is WAY too hard! I just can't do it." Wrong again! We have treated people who were working 14-16 hours a day. We found that they were able to use their time more effectively, because they had more physical and mental energy as a consequence of their nutrition, exercise, and lifestyle changes. They also had improvement in their brain function, leading to a greater sense of accomplishment and satisfaction. They were actually able to better balance their work, family, and play time, and they were more productive and happier than ever before.

Although it's best at this stage of the 20/20 LifeStyles plan not to dine out, for some of you that may not be possible. Initially, dining out will be a true test of your ability to accept, respect, and love yourself. Remember, in order to respect yourself, you need to respect your body, and that means showing yourself love by eating the healthy foods that will bring your body back to health and fitness. If dining out is necessary, here are some tips how you can dine out and still stay on your Stage 1 nutrition plan.

Before dining out, make sure you've eaten all of your Stage 1 meals and snacks on time throughout the day. Going out to eat when you're very hungry is a very bad idea. Next, think about what you're going to eat before you get to the restaurant. Make sure you'll be keeping to your Stage 1 nutrition plan of protein, fat, and one serving of berries.

A serving of meat or fish is about the size of a deck of cards or the palm of your hand.

If you're asked about a drink, have sparkling water with a twist of lemon or lime. Volunteer to be the designated driver to save you from having alcohol. In Stage 1, your body is detoxifying and increasing your metabolism's ability to burn more calories. Alcohol will stop that process and stop your weight loss. We'll talk more about alcohol in Chapter 10.

Don't open the menu! You know what you can eat and have already planned your meal, so just order it.

Order a 6 ounce filet mignon or 6 ounces of salmon or some other fish. Be sure to tell the waiter that you want it prepared without butter, oil, or sauces. That will give you both the protein and the fat you need for the meal. But now comes the hard part. The waiter will ask you about potatoes and other side dishes. Because you've decided to respect and love your body, you will reply, "None, thank you, I'm saving room for a serving of berries for dessert."

In Concept #10, we talked about assertiveness, and here's a place where you may have to use some. Someone in your group may say, "Oh, come on, have a drink with the rest of us," or "I guess you're on another diet," or "I have too many French fries, why don't you have some?"

Just say, "No, thank you" to the food and drink offers, and to the diet criticisms, say, "Yes, I want to live to see my kids grow up." That should quiet them down (26).

Here's an interesting test: Try to remember what you ate the last time that you dined out. You'll probably have difficulty remembering. This proves it's just not that important, but what you put into your body today is very important, because you are on the way to the new you.

We have more than 10,000 success stories-people who have tried the 20/20 LifeStyles program, loved it, and completed it. Try it. We believe you'll love it too.

---

26. See videos on Dining Right under Lifestyle series in Appendix J.

CHAPTER 10

LEARNING ABOUT YOUR BODY

STAGE 2

Congratulations, the hardest part is now behind you! The first week is the most rigorous and challening part of the meal plan, and you've succeeded. You probably never knew you could get so excited about eating vegetables, either.

At this point, you should be getting a bit more comfortable with your meal plan. If you're still feeling hesitant or anxious about the plan for any reason, you need to find out why. Over the years, we've identified some likely causes of continued discomfort. The main one is likely what you eat or drink. If you've eaten ANYTHING off-plan, that's probably what's holding up your adjustment. If you think that's the case, stick to plan 100 percent this week and see if your comfort level improves. If, on the other hand, you've been true to your food plan but are still experiencing discomfort, read on.

Foods are often advertised as being "diet," "low fat," "low sugar," "light," "lite," etc. But that's deceptive. They're actually fat builders loaded with sugar, fat, and salt. Sugar, fat, and salt work directly on the pleasure center of your brain-the reward center[27]. They increase the production of neurotransmitters that do two things. First, they make you feel better emotionally. Second, they increase your focus on that particular food, which leads to intense cravings. So read the ingredients!

27. David Kessler, MD, *The End of Overeating*, Rodale Books, April 2009.

If your grandmother wouldn't know what an ingredient is, or if you need an advanced degree in chemistry to identify the component, don't put it in your body [28].

Now let's talk about a really big problem for many of the people we've seen: ALCOHOL. Initially we allowed our program participants to have one glass of wine per week, but we found that those who had even one glass lost less weight or no weight that week. We just couldn't believe that one glass of wine could do that, so we suspected they were being less than completely honest in their meal tracker. But time after time our patients swore they were being totally honest.

This led us to believe that, with regard to alcohol, calories are not the issue. We believe that with alcohol in your system, a compound is created that gives your body a signal that it's in a high-energy state, or that there's an abundance of fuel in your system. And regardless of the calories in the alcoholic beverage you've had, your body switches over to the metabolic processes associated with storing energy. That's right, fat production. Fat production caused by consuming alcohol increases the circulating fatty acids in your blood and increases stored fat in your liver.

It's simple: If you want to succeed, avoid alcohol while completing this plan.

Your body is too important, and that glass of wine just isn't worth it! We'll discuss how to add alcohol back into your diet later, when we discuss maintenance. You can look as much as you like, but you will NOT find alcohol on our meal plan. If that's a problem for you, then you are making alcohol more important to you than your health, and you'd best examine your priorities. If you can't stop drinking during the course of this plan, you will simply not be successful at losing and maintaining your weight. If you find that not drinking during the course

28. See Reward Center videos under Nutrition in Appendix J.

of this plan is more difficult than you thought, you may need to talk to a counselor in your area who understands issues around alcohol.

If you can't seem to find a good support partner, it might be best to get the help of a counselor who is knowledgeable about the difficulties involved in weight loss and weight maintenance. Or, if you live in the Puget Sound Area, contact one of our counselors at: www.proclub.com/Wellness/Counseling

We hope that Stage 1 got your weight loss off to an excellent start. So, what's a good target? Your goal should be 1-2 percent of your body weight per week. For a 150-pound individual, a weekly loss of 1½ to 3 pounds would be right on track.

Stage 2 will bring a burst of flavor, color, and texture into your meal plan with the introduction of vegetables. Along with the increased variety, these colorful foods are great sources of vitamins, minerals, and fiber. At about 15 calories per serving, nonstarchy vegetables will increase the volume of your meals, with little impact on your daily caloric intake. Nonstarchy vegetables are those vegetables other than corn, peas, potatoes, sweet potatoes, and winter squash (we will discuss these in Stage 7). The starchy vegetables-corn, peas, potatoes, sweet potatoes, winter squash-don't figure in this phase of the plan. The 20/20 LifeStyles plan recommends 3 or more servings of nonstarchy vegetables at both lunch and dinner.

The only thing that changes with Stage 2 are the vegetables. The protein, berries, and healthy fats still remain unchanged. We recommend

3 servings of vegetables at lunch and at dinner. If this seems like too much, start with 2 servings and work your way up. For this week, salad dressings will be considered a fat serving. Include only those dressings with less than 6 grams of fat per serving. Make sure you read the label to determine portion size. The quantity you use will vary between different salad dressings, depending on the amount of fat in the dressing. For some dressings, the quantity will be 1 tablespoon, while for others the quantity may be 2 tablespoons. For more information, look at the dressings/sauces guidelines under the Stage 2 shopping list and Appendix E.

The most important rule with salad dressing is to always get your salads with dressing on the side. A good way to use salad dressing with your salad is to dip the fork in the salad dressing before you use the fork to pick up your bite of salad. We call this the fork trick, giving you the pleasant taste of the salad dressing while helping you consume less dressing and fewer calories.

Vegetables do contain carbohydrates, but their carbohydrate content is so much lower than that of grains or legumes that we put them in their own category. Vegetables are always your safe food. Don't worry about eating too many; no one ever gained weight from munching on too many cucumbers at lunch.

Embrace variety this week. Add a vegetable like bell peppers or zucchini to an egg-white scramble in the morning, or use spaghetti squash as a replacement for pasta in a traditional spaghetti meal[29]. You'll be eating vegetables at mealtimes for the rest of your life, so get creative!

For the rest of the plan and the rest of your new healthy life, lean protein and vegetables will compose the majority of your meals.

29. *See recipe in Appendix H.*

We like to think about Stage 2 as the meal plan foundation, or "home base."

Not only is Stage 2 great for weight loss as you begin the plan, it can also be used as a detox or reboot week.

If at any point in your plan you feel as if your meal plan is deviating, your body is out of balance, or weight is creeping back on, go back to Stage 2. That way you can refocus your attention on lean protein and vegetables. With the addition of vegetables, Stage 2 will meet all of your body's nutritional needs.

You may stay on Stage 2 as long as you like. The goal is to get comfortable with the protein and vegetable structure of this meal plan, as these two foods will be the bulk of your meals for the rest of your life. Many of our most successful participants have stayed on Stage 2 for many weeks, even months. They found that Stage 2 kept them fully satiated, the simple structure of the meals made meal planning easy, and their weight came off rapidly. Getting through this stage is not a race, so plan on staying at Stage 2 for the majority of your weight-loss journey. As a general rule, for every 15 pounds you plan to lose, remain on Stage 2 for one week.

Remember, Stage 2 sets your body back into balance, because it consists of the same food groups that the human body has adapted to for more than 10,000 years. Stage 2 eliminates hunger, because you'll be eating foods your body was designed to eat.

Dining out gets much easier in Stage 2. You can order a salad with dressing on the side, plus all the nonstarchy vegetables you want, steamed without butter, oil, or sauces. Remember to ask how much protein comes with the meal, because it's also important to make sure your salad or dish comes with a 4-6 ounce protein serving sufficient to keep you satiated. And, if you feel like it, you can still have a 1 cup serving of berries for dessert.

This plan will be the basis for your dining out until you have reached your goal weight and started your maintenance plan.

MEAL PLAN: THE BASICS

Stage 2 adds nonstarchy vegetables to your meal plan.

Serving Size:

- 3 or more servings of nonstarchy vegetables at lunch and at dinner.
- Leafy vegetables and salad greens, 1 serving = 1½ cups.
- Nonstarchy or green vegetables, 1 serving = ½ cup raw or cooked

1 serving of nonstarchy vegetables = approximately 15-30 calories.

SHOPPING LIST: VEGETABLES

Leafy Greens (1 serving = 1½ cups)

☐ Lettuce - Romaine, red, green leaf, Bibb, escarole

☐ Arugula

☐ Endive

☐ Spinach

Nonstarchy or Green Vegetables (1 serving= ½ cup)

☐ Artichoke

☐ Asparagus

- ☐ Broccoli*

- ☐ Brussels sprouts

- ☐ Bok choy

- ☐ Collards, mustard, or kale greens

- ☐ Green beans

- ☐ Zucchini*

Others *(1 serving= ½ cup)*

☐ Bean sprouts*	☐ Leeks
☐ Beets	☐ Mushrooms
☐ Bell peppers	☐ Onions
☐ Cabbage	☐ Radishes
☐ Carrots*	☐ Scallions
☐ Cauliflower	☐ Tomatoes
☐ Celery	☐ Water chestnuts
☐ Cucumber	☐ Spaghetti squash or yellow squash
☐ Eggplant	
☐ Jicama	

* These vegetables are high in fiber. Try to include at least one serving of a high-fiber vegetable each day.

Avoid juice, corn, peas, potatoes, yams, sweet potatoes, and winter squash due to their high starch content.

DRESSINGS AND SAUCES

Sauces, dressings or marinades are not required items on your meal plan. But if you would like to include a salad dressing, or marinade for your meat, these items will count as your fat serving for the meal. Make sure to read nutrition labels; salad dressings can range from 30 calories for a 2 tablespoon serving to 100 calories for 1 tablespoon. Fats are essential for satiety, but with fats as with all foods, moderation is the key. Follow the guidelines below to make sure your dressing is low in sugar, fat, and salt.

Refer to nutrition labels to determine serving size. Only include one serving of dressing with your meal, and always use the fork trick. Make sure to measure all dressings before you use them. When including a dressing, sauce, or marinade, only use items that follow these guidelines per serving:

Less than 6 grams sugar
Less than 6 grams fat
Less than 400 milligrams sodium

If you decide to use a fat-free dressing or a fat-free tomato or marinara sauce, continue to make sure they fit within the sugar and salt guidelines listed above. Lastly, limit these items to one serving per meal (servings determined by the amount given on the nutrition label) and continue to include your fat serving with the meal.

* For Stage 2, avoid dressings with yogurt or cheese in the ingredients. These items will be added back in Stage 3.

Marinades

- ☐ A1: Marinade
- ☐ Lawry's: Mexican Chili & Lime, Caribbean Jerk, Lemon Pepper, Steak & Chop, Baja Chipotle Mesquite, Havana Garlic & Lime, Italian Garlic Steak
- ☐ Masa's: Gourmet Curry Coconut, Thai Peanut Sauce

Soy Sauce *(less than 550 mg per serving of sodium)*

- ☐ Bragg Liquid Aminos (found near the soy sauces in the grocery store)
- ☐ Kroger: Lite Soy Sauce
- ☐ Yamasa: Less Salt Soy Sauce

Mayonnaise

- ☐ Hellmann's: Reduced Fat
- ☐ Kraft: Fat Free, Light

Tomato Sauce

- ☐ Emeril's: Kicked Up Tomato
- ☐ Muir Glen: All varieties

Salad Dressings

- ☐ Annie's Naturals: Lite Raspberry Vinaigrette, Tuscany Italian, Lite Gingerly Vinaigrette, Lite Honey Mustard Vinaigrette
- ☐ Trader Joe's: Champagne Pear Vinaigrette, Asian Spicy
- ☐ Kraft: Light Done Right Italian, Light Done Right Raspberry Vinaigrette, Fat Free Honey Dijon, Fat Free Zesty Italian, Zesty Italian, Sundried Tomato Vinaigrette
- ☐ Newman's Own Lights: Italian Dressing, Balsamic Vinaigrette,
- ☐ Lime Vinaigrette, Raspberry & Walnut

STAGE 2
Women 1,100-1,400 calories

BREAKFAST	CALORIES	FAT (g)
4 ounces very lean protein	140	0-4
2 heart-healthy fat servings *(see list for options)*	90	10
1 cup berries	80	0
OR		
Breakfast Shake Alternatives		

LUNCH	CALORIES	FAT (g)
4 ounces very lean/lean protein	140-220	0-12
1 heart-healthy fat servings *(add to very lean protein only)*	45	5
3 or more servings nonstarchy vegetables	45	0
1 cup berries	80	0

SNACK *(1 per day between lunch and dinner)*	CALORIES	FAT (g)
2 ounces very lean protein plus 1 cup berries	130	0-2
20/20 LifeStyles High Protein Dry Powder Shake plus 1 cup berries *(NO peanut butter)*	260	0

DINNER	CALORIES	FAT (g)
4 ounces very lean/lean protein	140-220	0-12
1 heart-healthy fat servings *(add to very lean protein only)*	45	5
3 or more servings nonstarchy vegetables	45	0
20/20 LifeStyles High Protein Dry Powder Shake plus 1 cup berries *(NO peanut butter)*	260	0

SAMPLE MENU

DAY 1

BREAKFAST:

- 20/20 LifeStyles High Protein Dry Powder Shake

- 1 tablespoon peanut butter

- 1 cup blackberries

LUNCH:

- 4 ounces pork tenderloin baked with 1 tablespoon pork marinade *(try Stubb's)*

- 1½ cups broccoli

- 1 cup strawberries

SNACK:

- 20/20 LifeStyles Protein Bar

DINNER:

- 4 ounces chicken breast

- Salad containing:

    ~ 1½ cups chopped romaine lettuce

    ~ ¼ cup chopped carrots

    ~ ¼ cup chopped tomatoes

    ~ 2 tablespoons low-fat salad dressing

- 20/20 LifeStyles High Protein Dry Powder Shake plus 1 cup berries *(NO peanut butter)*

DAY 2

BREAKFAST:

- Using 2 teaspoons olive oil, make an omelet of:

    ~ 1 cup Egg Beaters

    ~ ½ cup chopped green or red bell peppers

    ~ ¼ cup chopped tomato

- 1 cup strawberries

LUNCH:

- 4 ounces baked salmon with splash of lemon juice and 1 teaspoon chopped dill

- 1½ cup steamed green beans

- 1 cup raspberries

SNACK:

- - 2 ounces low-sodium turkey jerky

- - 1 cup blueberries

DINNER:

- - Cook a mock spaghetti sauce, using 1 teaspoon oil, of:

  - ~ 4 ounces very lean ground beef

  - ~ ½ cup low-sodium pasta sauce

  - ~ ½ cup chopped onions

  - ~ ½ cup mushroom

  - ~ Italian seasoning for flavor

- - Pour over:

  - ~ 1 cup cooked spaghetti squash

- - 20/20 LifeStyles High Protein Dry Powder Shake plus 1 cup berries (*NO peanut butter*)

DAY 3

BREAKFAST:

- - Using 1 teaspoon oil, scramble:

  - ~ 2 ounces turkey sausage

  - ~ 1 large whole egg

  - ~ 2 egg whites

- - 1 cup marionberries

SNACK:

- ½ cup shelled edamame
- 1 cup mixed berries

LUNCH:

- 4 ounces grilled chicken breast
- 6 almonds
- 1 cup steamed broccoli mixed with ½ cup steamed cauliflower
- 1 cup strawberries

DINNER:

- 4 ounces baked cod fillet
- Salad made with:
    - 1½ cups cooked spinach plus 1 teaspoon roasted garlic
    - ½ cup cooked carrots
    - ½ cup chopped cucumber
- 20/20 LifeStyles High Protein Dry Powder Shake + 1 cup berries
(NO peanut butter)

STAGE 2

Men 1,300-1,700 calories

BREAKFAST	CALORIES	FAT (g)
4 ounces very lean protein	140	0-4
2 heart-healthy fat servings *(see list for options)*	90	10
1 cup berries	80	0
OR		
Breakfast Shake Alternatives		

LUNCH	CALORIES	FAT (g)
6 ounces very lean/lean protein	210-330	0-18
1 heart-healthy fat servings *(add to very lean protein only)*	45	5
3 or more servings nonstarchy vegetables	45	0
1 cup berries	80	0

SNACK *(2 per day between lunch and dinner): Choose ONE of these options for your snack.*	CALORIES	FAT (g)
2 ounces very lean protein plus 1 cup berries	130	0-2
20/20 LifeStyles High Protein Dry Powder Shake plus 1 cup berries *(NO peanut butter)*	260	0

DINNER	CALORIES	FAT (g)
6 ounces very lean/lean protein	210-330	0-18
1 heart-healthy fat servings *(add to very lean protein only)*	45	5
3 or more servings nonstarchy vegetables	45	0
20/20 LifeStyles High Protein Dry Powder Shake plus 1 cup berries *(NO peanut butter)*	260	0

Because starch rapidly turns to sugar in the body, you need to think of starch and sugar as synonymous.

Starchy vegetables will be added in Stage 7. They are higher in calories and much higher in carbohydrates than nonstarchy vegetables. Because of the increase in carbohydrates, starchy vegetables can often cause hunger cravings. For Stage 2, only include the vegetables on the list.

For some exciting and delicious ways to prepare vegetables, see Appendix F.

SAMPLE MENUS

DAY 1

BREAKFAST:

- 20/20 LifeStyles High Protein Dry Powder Shake

- 1 tablespoon peanut butter

- 1 cup blueberries

SNACK:

- 20/20 LifeStyles Protein Bar

LUNCH:

- 6 ounces pork tenderloin baked with 1 tablespoon pork marinade *(try Stubb's)*
- 1½ cup steamed broccoli
- 1 cup strawberries

SNACK:

- 2 ounces low-sodium turkey jerky
- 1 cup blueberries

DINNER:

- 6 ounces baked chicken breast
- Salad made with:
    - 1½ cups romaine lettuce
    - ¼ cup chopped carrots
    - ¼ cup chopped tomatoes
    - 2 tablespoons low-fat salad dressing
- 20/20 LifeStyles High Protein Dry Powder Shake plus 1 cup berries *(NO peanut butter)*

DAY 2

BREAKFAST:

- Using 1 teaspoon oil, make an omelet of:
    - ~ 1 cup Egg Beaters
    - ~ ½ cup chopped green or red bell pepper
    - ~ ¼ cup chopped tomato
- 1 cup strawberries

SNACK:

- 2 ounces low-sodium deli turkey
- 1 cup strawberries

LUNCH:

- 6 ounces baked salmon with splash of lemon juice plus 1 teaspoon chopped dill
- 1 cup steamed green beans
- 1 cup raspberries

SNACK:

- ½ cup shelled edamame
- 1 cup mixed berries

DINNER:

- Using 1 teaspoon oil, cook a mock spaghetti sauce with:

    ~ 6 ounces very lean ground beef

    ~ ½ cup low-sodium pasta sauce

    ~ ½ cup chopped onions

    ~ ½ cup mushrooms

    ~ Italian seasoning for flavor

- Pour the mixture over: 1 cup cooked spaghetti squash

- 20/20 LifeStyles High Protein Dry Powder Shake plus 1 cup berries *(NO peanut butter)*

DAY 3

BREAKFAST:

- Using 1 teaspoon olive oil, scramble:

    ~ 2 ounces low-sodium turkey sausage

    ~ 1 large egg

    ~ 2 egg whites

- 1 cup mixed berries

SNACK:

- 2 ounces turkey breast

- 1 cup raspberries

LUNCH:

- 6 ounces baked chicken breast
- 6 almonds
- 1 cup steamed broccoli mixed with ½ cup steamed cauliflower
- 1 cup strawberries

SNACK:

- 2 ounces grilled chicken strips
- 1 cup blackberries

DINNER:

- 6 ounces cod fillet, baked with 1 teaspoon oil
- Make a salad with:
    - 1½ cups spinach cooked with 1 teaspoon roasted garlic
    - ½ cup cooked carrots
    - ½ cup chopped cucumber
- 20/20 LifeStyles High Protein Dry Powder Shake plus 1 cup berries *(NO peanut butter)*

EXERCISE PLAN: MOVING UP

At this point, if you aren't used to exercise, you may feel a little fatigued after working out. That's normal, and it will pass as your body adapts to your routine and becomes more fit. After just a few weeks, exercise will begin to give you more energy, make you mentally sharper, and help with any sleep problems you're having.

Be sure to log your exercise in your meal tracker. It's great to look back and see your progress. If you're diligent about the exercise portion of this plan, we'll give you the best toy you've ever had-your body! Your body will become a tool for such new activities as skiing, hiking, snowboarding, or even running. It will also become something you're proud to show off at events and gatherings. A healthy, fit body is a public example of your hard work, a reflection of your lifestyle. Be diligent with your exercise routine, and the results will astound and please you.

EXERCISE WILL BE AS FOLLOWS

Level 1: Low fitness- We will increase the intensity of your exercise slowly. Increasing too rapidly can cause stress on ligaments, tendons, and joints and lead to injury. Injury means a significant delay in your plan and nobody wants that. So don't try to set any records here. Follow the recommended directions. Try walking at a moderate speed for 30 minutes at least five days per week. Try to increase your pace to get close to your minimum optimum heart rate (55-65 percent of your maximum heart rate). At this point, you will need to buy a heart-rate monitor. See Chapter 9, Stage 1, under Moderate Fitness for how to buy a heart-rate monitor and how to calculate your optimum heart rates.

Level 2: Moderate fitness- High-speed walking for 30 minutes, then running five minutes at least five days per week. If running is difficult for you, then just continue high-speed walking for the additional five minutes. You should keep your heart rate at the optimum level (65-85 percent of your maximum).

Level 3: High fitness- Running for 35 minutes at least five days per week. Heart rate at optimum level.

Now, in your second week, your body is going to begin to try to protect itself against weight loss. One of the main ways it will do this is by decreasing your nonexercise activity. As mentioned earlier, we call this non-exercise activity thermogenesis, or NEAT. Most normal Americans average 5,000 steps per day. Your body will try to decrease this to 4,000, 3,000 or even 2,500 steps per day. You must make a conscious effort to keep your steps up at 5,000-6,000 steps per day. The only way you can do this is with a pedometer. Pedometers are very easy to purchase and are a crucial tool for your continued success.

Keep in mind that these 5,000 steps do not include the steps you get while exercising. Your pedometer should be removed during exercise. When you get home at the end of your day and you find your steps are low, you'll need to go for a walk to get your steps up to 5,000 or more; otherwise your weight loss will slow down.

Another way to speed up weight loss is to increase steps beyond the 5,000-6,000 range. Many of our patients walk 10,000 or more steps per day to speed up their weight loss.

LIFESTYLE PLAN: FEELINGS

Many of you eat due to feelings. Loneliness, boredom, anger, depression, and frustration are popular offenders, but joy and celebration are problems for some as well. In this section, we talk about two factors that are a big problem-stress and depression. Stress and depression actually resemble each other, both from a clinical perspective and in your body's chemical response. For our purposes, the villain is the hormone cortisol, which your adrenal gland produces when you're stressed or depressed. Cortisol does a number of things to your body, all bad. Cortisol causes insulin resistance, fat storage, weight gain, and cell ageing. It also makes you very hungry! Not only do stress and depression cause you to produce excess cortisol, but if you're stressed, those around you will also produce excess cortisol in their own bodies within 15 minutes of being in contact with you. You've become a walking weapon of mass destruction.

We realize that everyone is different, and each of you has a different tolerance to triggers that cause stress or depression. Many of you will initially experience stress, depression, or both, but after four to six weeks of good nutrition, exercise, and lifestyle change, these problems will resolve. But if they don't, then those are instances where you may need additional help.

The first step in getting a handle on these life and diet destroyers is being 100 percent honest with yourself. Denial of illness is a well-known phenomenon in the medical field. People just don't want to admit they have a problem. In the worst cases, this can cause severe illness and death. In the 20/20 LifeStyles plan, denial causes failure. Those family members and friends closest to you can help you through this denial. Ask them if they believe that you're stressed or depressed. Often, things you think you've been concealing are quite obvious to those who know you best.

If you find that you really are in denial, it's essential for you to take action if you expect to have long-term success with your weight and your health. Sit down with a paper and pencil, a laptop or PC, and write down what you perceive as the problems in your life. Now, write down the problem you really didn't want to write down-you know, the one that raises your anxiety when you think about it: the job that needs changing, the relationship that needs changing, the children that are out of control, the finances that seem hopeless.

Next, you'll need to get some support. Making scary changes is hard if you're making them alone. The support of others makes these changes possible. If you find you can't move beyond this point, you'll require additional outside help. Talk to a counselor or psychologist in your area, or if you live in the Puget Sound area, contact one of our counselors: www.proclub.com/Wellness/Counseling

Admitting you need help is always difficult. You may feel that if you have to get help, you must be badly broken. That's not the case. Think of a psychologist or counselor as a consultant. They'll help you manage difficult parts of your life, in the same way that a business will hire a financial or marketing consultant to help manage difficult parts of their enterprise. The smart business asks for help, the not-so-smart business goes broke.

CHAPTER 11

LEARNING ABOUT YOUR BODY

STAGE 3 AND STAGE 4

Welcome to Stage 3! At this point in the meal plan, you should be very comfortable with the protein and vegetable structure of your meals. As we said, you can live the rest of your life on protein and vegetables. So, moving on to Stage 3 is optional.

Foods are classified into three macronutrient categories: protein, fat, or carbohydrate. As you move forward through this plan, you can determine how to classify a food by knowing the main macronutrient content of that food. The new foods for Stage 3 include low-fat cheese, low-fat or nonfat cottage cheese, and nonfat plain Greek yogurt. All these items are classified as proteins.

Low-fat cheeses, low-fat and nonfat cottage cheeses, and nonfat plain Greek yogurt are considered proteins, if the number of grams of protein in the food is at least double the grams of carbohydrate.

For cheeses, only include items with less than 6 grams of fat per ounce. Low-fat or nonfat cottage cheese and nonfat plain Greek yogurts may be included, but not fruit-flavored Greek yogurt. All these items are in the protein family as well.

For Stage 3, you'll notice that the lean and very lean proteins, 1 cup berry servings, and heart-healthy fats and vegetables remain unchanged from Stage 2. Protein and vegetables are still the stars of the show in regard to your plate.

In Stage 3, you should include 0-2 servings of the dairy-based items listed above per day. Do not exceed the recommendation of 2 servings per day. We recommend limiting intake of low-fat cheeses, cottage cheese, and Greek yogurt because these items are dairy products, and dairy products can slow down or halt weight loss for some individuals.

When you measure the foods added in Stage 3, make sure you measure them properly. If you want ¼ cup low-fat cheese, don't pack it down. A ¼ cup serving of either cottage cheese or a ½ cup serving of nonfat plain Greek yogurt should be level, not heaping.

We consider these items proteins, so when using them at a meal you must decrease your protein serving by 1 ounce. For example: 3 ounces of chicken plus ¼ cup of shredded low-fat cheese will be the equivalent of your 4 ounce protein serving for the meal. This way you can keep calories within range yet allow for more variety in your meals.

Because the taste of nonfat plain Greek yogurt is very tart, when using it as one of your snacks we highly recommend that you mix your ½ cup serving of plain Greek yogurt with 1cup thawed frozen berries. The natural sugars of the berries infuse with the tart plain Greek yogurt to produce a sweet, delectable snack. Two light Laughing Cow wedges (1 serving) melt wonderfully over vegetables, and ¼ cup low-fat shredded cheese can be a great addition to a salad. As we pointed out in Stage 2, variety within meals is your friend. You'll want to build a meal plan full of foods you enjoy. Not only will variety and tasty meals help you lose weight successfully, those two assets will help you keep it off!

Lastly, for some individuals, dairy products can cause digestive problems and slow down or completely halt weight loss. Be mindful of the scale this week, and know that if your weight loss slows down or you experience stomach discomfort, dairy-based products in Stage 3 could be the reason. So, if you find this happens to you, remove all cheese, nonfat Greek yogurt, and low-fat and nonfat cottage cheese from your meal plan during your weight-loss stages. Keep all dairy products out of your meal plan until you reach your desired weight. Once you have reached your goal weight, add these items back in moderation. If you find you gain weight or experience abdominal pain or bloating, take dairy products out of your diet forever.

It is not uncommon for certain populations to use dairy foods sparingly, if at all. Asian cultures, for example have some of the lowest dairy consumption in the world. If your traditional diet does not include dairy-based products, don't feel obligated to add any new foods in Stage 3. Other cultures may use dairy-based products, such as yogurt, in cooking. To ensure optimal weight loss, if you do decide to add some low-fat cheese, nonfat plain Greek yogurt, or low-fat or nonfat cottage cheese to your meal plan, keep your servings of these foods to a maximum of 2 per day.

STAGE 3

MEAL PLAN: ADDING VARIETY

Stage 3 includes low-fat cheese, nonfat plain Greek yogurt, low-fat and nonfat cottage cheese, counting these items in the protein category.

Servings: 0-2 servings per day for men and women.

Serving Sizes:

- Low-fat cheese: 1 serving = 1 ounce or ¼ cup shredded

    - 1 ounce of cubed or nonshredded cheese = 1 slice the size of a Post-It note, or a chunk the size of 2 dominoes

- Nonfat plain Greek yogurt: 1 serving = ½ cup

- Low-fat and nonfat cottage cheese: 1 serving = ¼ cup

Calorie range: 35-90 calories per serving

SHOPPING LIST: LOW-FAT CHEESE

Cheddar

☐ Trader Joe's Reduced Fat Cheddar

☐ Trader Joe's Sliced Lite Cheddar

☐ Trader Joe's Reduced Fat Celtic Cheddar

☐ Cabot 75 percent Light Cheddar

☐ Cabot 50 percent Light Cheddar

Mozzarella

☐ Kraft 2 percent Shredded Mozzarella

String cheese

- ☐ Frigo Light Cheese Heads (1 stick)
- ☐ Kraft Light String-Ums (1 stick)
- ☐ Sargento Light (1 stick)

Swiss

- ☐ Jarlsberg Lite Swiss
- ☐ Heavenly Light Swiss
- ☐ Laughing Cow Light
- ☐ Creamy Swiss Original (2 wedges = 1 serving)
- ☐ Laughing Cow
- ☐ Mini Babybel Light (1 round piece = 1 serving)
- ☐ Kraft 2 percent (3/4 ounce slice)

Colby

- ☐ Kraft Reduced Fat

Monterey Jack

- ☐ Kraft 2 percent

Parmesan (regular): Use as a condiment for flavor

- ☐ Shredded/grated (2 tablespoons)

Feta

- ☐ Athenos Reduced Fat Feta
- ☐ President Fat Free Crumbled Feta

Ricotta

- ☐ Fat-Free or Low-Fat varieties (¼ cup)

Brie

- ☐ Trader Joe's Light Brie

Blue cheese

☐ Treasure Cave Reduced-Fat Blue Cheese

Cottage cheese

☐ Fat-free or low-fat varieties (¼ cup)

High-protein yogurt

Criteria: Protein should be equal to or greater than twice the carbohydrate. Serving size = ½ cup

☐ Fage Total 0 percent

☐ Chobani 0 percent Plain

☐ OIKOS 0 percent Organic Greek Yogurt

☐ Voskos 0 percent Plain Greek Yogurt

☐ Trader Joe's Greek Style 0 percent Plain Yogurt

☐ Siggi's Plain Nonfat

STAGE 3

Women 1,100-1,400 calories

BREAKFAST	CALORIES	FAT (g)
4 ounces very lean protein	140	0-4
2 heart-healthy fat servings *(see list for options)*	90	10
1 cup berries	80	0
OR		
Breakfast Shake Alternatives		

LUNCH	CALORIES	FAT (g)
4 ounces very lean/lean protein OR 3 ounces very lean or lean protein plus 1 ounce cheese	140-220	0-12
1 heart-healthy fat servings *(add to very lean protein only)*	45	5
3 or more servings nonstarchy vegetables	45	0
1 cup berries	80	0

SNACK *(1 per day between lunch and dinner)*	CALORIES	FAT (g)
1 cup nonfat or low-fat plain Greek yogurt plus 1 cup berries	130-150	0-2
2 low fat-string cheeses plus 1 cup berries	180-200	5
2 ounces very lean protein plus 1 cup berries	130	0-2
20/20 LifeStyles High Protein Dry Powder Shake plus 1 cup berries *(NO peanut butter)*	260	0

DINNER	CALORIES	FAT (g)
4 ounces very lean/lean protein OR 3 ounces very lean or lean protein plus 1 ounce cheese	140-220	0-12
1 heart-healthy fat servings *(add to very lean protein only)*	45	5
3 or more servings nonstarchy vegetables	45	0
20/20 LifeStyles High Protein Dry Powder Shake plus 1 cup berries *(NO peanut butter)*	260	0

SAMPLE MENU

DAY 1

BREAKFAST:

- 20/20 LifeStyles High Protein Dry Powder Shake

- 1 tablespoon peanut butter

- 1 cup blueberries

LUNCH:

- 4 ounces baked chicken breast

- Make a salad with:

~ 1½ cups baby spinach

~ ½ cup diced carrots

~ ½ cup chopped tomatoes

~ 2 tablespoon low-fat salad dressing

- 1 cup strawberries

SNACK :

- 20/20 LifeStyles Protein Bar

DINNER:

- 4 ounces grilled salmon

- 1½ cups steamed asparagus with 1 tablespoon fresh Parmesan cheese

- 20/20 LifeStyles High Protein Dry Powder Shake plus 1 cup berries *(NO peanut butter)*

DAY 2

BREAKFAST:

- 1 cup nonfat plain Greek yogurt with 1 cup thawed frozen raspberries

- 1 tablespoon peanut butter

LUNCH:

- 1-2 green bell peppers, halved and seeded

- In 1 teaspoon olive oil, cook:

   ⁓ 4 ounces very lean ground beef

   ⁓ ½ cup chopped onion

   ⁓ Add ½ cup low-sodium marinara sauce to meat mixture

   ⁓ Stuff peppers with mixture

- 1 cup blueberries

SNACK:

- 2 ounces low-sodium deli turkey

- 1 cup strawberries

DINNER:

- 4 ounces baked pork tenderloin

- 1 cup steamed broccoli

- 20/20 LifeStyles High Protein Dry Powder Shake plus 1 cup berries *(NO peanut butter)*

DAY 3

BREAKFAST:

- With 1 teaspoon oil, scramble:

  ~ 3 egg whites

  ~ 1 ounce low-sodium ham

  ~ Add ¼ cup shredded low-fat cheddar cheese for flavor

- 1 cup strawberries

LUNCH:

- 4 ounces chicken breast, baked with 1 teaspoon oil

- Dash no-sodium seasoning for flavor

- 1 cup steamed green beans

- ½ cup diced tomatoes

- 1 cup raspberries

SNACK:

- 1 low-fat string cheese stick

- 1 cup blueberries

DINNER:

- 4 ounces grilled filet mignon

- ½ cup steamed zucchini

- ½ cup steamed yellow squash

- 20/20 LifeStyles High Protein Dry Powder Shake plus 1 cup berries *(NO peanut butter)*

STAGE 3

Men 1,300-1,700 calories

BREAKFAST	CALORIES	FAT (g)
4 ounces very lean protein	140	0-4
2 heart-healthy fat servings *(see list for options)*	90	10
1 cup berries	80	0
OR		
Breakfast Shake Alternatives		

LUNCH	CALORIES	FAT (g)
6 ounces very lean/lean protein OR 5 ounces very lean or lean protein plus 1 ounce cheese	210-330	0-18
1 heart-healthy fat servings *(add to very lean protein only)*	45	5
3 or more servings nonstarchy vegetables	45	0
1 cup berries	80	0

SNACK *(2 per day between lunch and dinner): Choose ONE of these options for your snack.*	CALORIES	FAT (g)
1 cup nonfat or low-fat plain Greek yogurt plus 1 cup berries	130-150	0-2
2 low fat-string cheeses plus 1 cup berries	180-200	5
2 ounces very lean protein plus 1 cup berries	130	0-2
20/20 LifeStyles High Protein Dry Powder Shake plus 1 cup berries *(NO peanut butter)*	260	0

DINNER	CALORIES	FAT (g)
6 ounces very lean/lean protein OR 5 ounces very lean or lean protein plus 1 ounce cheese	210-330	0-18
1 heart-healthy fat servings *(add to very lean protein only)*	45	5
3 or more servings nonstarchy vegetables	45	0
20/20 LifeStyles High Protein Dry Powder Shake plus 1 cup berries *(NO peanut butter)*	260	0

SAMPLE MENU

DAY 1

BREAKFAST:

- 20/20 LifeStyles High Protein Dry Powder Shake

- 1 tablespoon peanut butter

- 1 cup blackberries

SNACK:

- 2 ounces low-sodium turkey jerky

- 1 cup raspberries

LUNCH:

- 6 ounces chicken breast

- Salad made with:

~ 1½ cups baby spinach

- ½ cup diced carrots

- ½ cup chopped tomatoes

- ¼ cup low-fat goat cheese crumbles

- 2 tablespoons low-fat salad dressing

- 1 cup strawberries

SNACK:

- 20/20 LifeStyles Protein Bar

DINNER:

- 6 ounces grilled salmon

- 1½ cups steamed asparagus

- 20/20 LifeStyles High Protein Dry Powder Shake plus 1 cup berries *(NO peanut butter)*

DAY 2

BREAKFAST:

- 1 cup plain Greek yogurt

- 1 cup raspberries

- 2 tablespoons chopped almonds

SNACK:

- 2 ounces low-sodium deli ham

- 1 cup blueberries

LUNCH:

- Cook 6 ounces very lean ground beef

- Mix with ½ cup low-sodium marinara sauce

- Serve atop 1½ cups cooked spaghetti squash

- 1 cup blueberries

- 10 peanuts

SNACK:

- 2 ounces low-sodium deli turkey

- 1 cup strawberries

DINNER:

- 6 ounces baked pork tenderloin

- 1½ cups steamed broccoli

- 20/20 LifeStyles High Protein Dry Powder Shake plus 1 cup berries *(NO peanut butter)*

DAY 3

BREAKFAST:

- Using 1 teaspoon oil, scramble:

  ~ 4 egg whites

  ~ 1 ounce low-sodium diced ham

  ~ ¼ cup shredded low-fat cheese

SNACK:

- 1 ounce low-fat cheddar cheese

- 1 ounce low-sodium deli turkey

- 1 cup blueberries

LUNCH:

- 6 ounces chicken breast, cooked with 1 teaspoon oil

- Dash no-sodium-added seasoning for flavor

- 1 cup steamed green beans

- ½ cup diced tomatoes

- 1 cup raspberries

SNACK:

- ¾ cup shelled edamame

- 1 cup blueberries

DINNER:

- 6 ounces grilled filet mignon

- 1 cup steamed zucchini

- ½ cup steamed yellow squash

- 20/20 High Protein Dry Powder Shake plus 1 cup berries *(NO peanut butter)*

EXERCISE PLAN: FEELING THE CHANGE

Level 1: Low fitness- We can begin to increase the intensity of your workout a bit faster now. Your ligaments, tendons, muscles, and joints are getting stronger due to your previous weeks' workouts. Moderate- to high-speed walking for 45 minutes, at least five days per week. Try to increase your pace to reach minimum optimum heart rate (65 percent of your maximum).

Level 2: Moderate fitness- High-speed walking for 30 minutes, then running for 15 minutes, at least five days per week. If running is difficult for you, add an extra 15 minutes of high-speed walking; you may have to walk gradual hills to keep your heart rate up. You should keep your heart rate at optimum level (65-85 percent of your maximum).

Level 3: High fitness- Running for 45 minutes, at least five days per week. Start running gradual hills. Heart rate at optimum level (65-85 percent of your maximum).

All Levels: Make sure to pay attention to how your body is feeling and recovering after your exercise. It's normal to feel a little sore for a day or so, but chronic soreness is not normal. Make sure you continue to get enough rest and recovery time to avoid injury. You need to be sleeping a minimum of 7½ hours per night.

You must keep your steps at a high level to avoid having your NEAT decrease. Increase your pedometer steps to a minimum of 6,000 steps per day, and be sure to track your steps in your tracker. Start taking the stairs up instead of the elevator. Park on the far side of the parking lot and walk to the building. Get up during commercials while watching TV and walk around (avoiding the kitchen). If your job is sedentary, take a 2-minute break each hour to move around.

LIFESTYLE PLAN: TIME PLANNING

As the renowned physicist Albert Einstein noted, time is inflexible; it does not stretch, bend, or expand. Each day has 24 hours, and during that time, you must accomplish everything you have to do that day. Long ago, I noted in my medical practice how difficult it was to make appointments with retired patients, because they were so busy. This led me to become more aware of how we use time. The principle seems to be that no matter how much time you have available, you'll fill it up and usually overfill it.

You've decided you want to look better and feel better, and that takes time. Planning meals, exercising, taking time for yourself, and getting enough sleep takes time. Since your time is 100 percent full, and since Einstein told us you can't stretch it, that leaves only one option: You must give something up to make room for something else. This is the basic truth about time management; it involves extremely difficult decisions. Some of these decisions may be, "Do I work fewer hours and risk getting fired," or "Do I spend less time with my family and risk getting divorced," or "Do I spend less time at a hobby or activity I love and risk feeling deprived and unhappy?"

You will have to get creative to solve these dilemmas. You might consider taking your family with you when you exercise. You might also have the whole family participate in a sport such as hiking or snowboarding.

At work, you'll need to operate on a basis of knowledge, not fear. If you "only" work 45 hours per week, will you really lose your job or your next promotion? Talk to friends in the company and ask their opinion. Talk to your family about time and activities. Don't let your fears ruin your time plan.

Fortunately, as your body and mind become healthier, you'll naturally become more efficient and productive.

You'll get more done in less time.

You also need to differentiate between time and quality time. How many of your work hours are spent surfing the internet, chatting with associates, or on personal phone calls and text messages? How much of your family time is spent in front of the TV or the PC? If you're efficient in your use of time, you can get more for less, especially when your body and mind are healthy. One hour spent with your child having breakfast out on the weekend can be more valuable than eight hours working in the kitchen while your child watches TV.

From the beginning of this book, we've told you that there is no permanent change without a lifestyle change. Now we're telling you there is no lifestyle change without time planning.

STAGE 4

In Stage 4 you can introduce all fruits. The key to Stage 4 meals is serving size. For such whole fruits as apples, pears, and oranges, one serving is equivalent to a tennis-ball-size fruit. For such fruits as grapes or cut-up fruit, say melon or pineapple, one serving is ½ cup. Remember, measure out a level ½ cup, not heaping.

In Stage 1, we discussed that berries are in their own category because of their low carbohydrate content. We understand that berries are technically a fruit, but we consider them as a separate food group from the rest of the fruits introduced in Stage 4. Berries are their own food group and may be used in 1 cup servings. Other fruit may not. The rest of the fruits are higher in sugar, and you may only consume ½ cup of any of those at a time. If you exceed the ½ cup serving at one sitting, your hunger and cravings can return. At mealtimes, you may use 1 cup of berries for your carbohydrate serving, or substitute ½ cup fruit in their place.

> *To remember the difference between berries and other fruits: Berries are good; you can have twice as many. For the rest of the fruits, a half cup is plenty!*

In the past, you may have noticed that once you start to munch on some fruit such as grapes, you keep right on munching, without ever feeling full. This is because fruits are simple carbohydrates-in other words, a simple sugar. Simple sugars are broken down and absorbed in your body very rapidly. They provide fuel for your cells either to use immediately or to store for later use. While fruit is a great source of quick energy, it will not keep you satiated for a prolonged period of time.

Eating simple carbohydrates by themselves can cause a dramatic spike in your blood sugar soon after you eat them. The subsequent crash from that spike can cause hunger and cravings. To avoid this, don't eat more than ½ cup of fruit at a time, and always pair the fruit with two servings of a healthy fat or 2 ounces of protein. Protein and healthy fat break down in your body much more slowly than carbohydrates, so including protein or fat with all meals and snacks will keep you satiated. Healthy fat examples include 1 tablespoon of nut butter, 12 almonds, or ¼ avocado. Proteins you may pair with fruit include such items as two string cheeses, or 2 ounces of low-sodium deli meat. One apple (carbohydrate) the size of a tennis ball with ½ cup low-fat cottage cheese (protein) makes a great balanced 1:1 protein/carbohydrate snack.

So, from now on, remember: Never eat a carb alone. Always marry a carbohydrate with a protein or healthy fat.

When using frozen fruits, always choose unsweetened frozen fruits to be sure no sugar has been added. As for portions, you may substitute ½ cup unsweetened frozen fruit for ½ cup fresh fruit.

Notice that dried fruits and fruit juice are NOT included in the 20/20 LifeStyles meal plan. Dried fruits are much higher in calories and lower in overall volume than fresh fruits. Eating ½ cup of raisins yields 220 calories, where ½ cup of grapes yields 60! As for juice, your body doesn't recognize juice as a calorie-dense beverage. That's why drinking juice won't make you full.

From now on, think of juice as sugar, on account of its small volume and high calorie content.

A ½ cup serving of orange juice yields 60 calories and ½ gram of fiber, whereas a medium orange yields 60 calories and 3 grams of fiber. So, eat the orange; don't drink the juice. Eating whole fruits will always be a much healthier and more satisfying option than dried fruit or juices. That's why the 20/20 LifeStyles plan does not include fruit juices or dried fruits.

If you find that certain fruits trigger your hunger, don't include them in your meal plan. Your body can always get sufficient carbohydrates from berries. So, if introducing a new type of fruit makes you hungry, remove it and replace it with a cup of berries.

MEAL PLAN: AN APPLE A DAY

Stage 4 adds fruit to your meal plan.

Guidelines: 2-4 servings per day

Serving Size:

- 1 serving of fruit = ½ cup

- Whole fruits: 1 serving = a small fruit the size of a tennis ball

1 serving of fruit = 60 Calories

SHOPPING LIST: FRUIT

☐ Apple

☐ Apricot

☐ Banana (serving size is ½ medium)

☐ Blackberries

☐ Blueberries

☐ Boysenberries

☐ Cantaloupe

☐ Cherries

☐ Grapefruit

☐ Grapes

☐ Honeydew melon

☐ Kiwifruit

☐ Mango

☐ Marionberries

☐ Nectarine

☐ Orange

☐ Papaya

☐ Peach

☐ Pear

☐ Pineapple

☐ Plums

☐ Raspberries

☐ Strawberries

☐ Tangerines

☐ Watermelon

STAGE 4
Women 1,100-1,400 calories

BREAKFAST	CALORIES	FAT (g)
4 ounces very lean protein	140	0-4
2 heart-healthy fat servings *(see list for options)*	90	10
1 cup berries	80	0
OR		
Breakfast Shake Alternatives		

LUNCH	CALORIES	FAT (g)
4 ounces very lean/lean protein OR 3 ounces very lean or lean protein plus 1 ounce cheese	140-220	0-12
1 heart-healthy fat servings *(add to very lean protein only)*	45	5
3 or more servings nonstarchy vegetables	45	0
Choose one of the following		
1 cup berries OR ½ cup fruit	60-80	0

SNACK *(1 per day between lunch and dinner)*	CALORIES	FAT (g)
½ cup nonfat or low-fat cottage cheese plus ½ cup fruit	160-180	0-2
1 cup nonfat or low-fat plain Greek yogurt plus ½ cup fruit	140-170	0-4
2 ounces very lean protein plus 1 cup berries	130	0-2
20/20 LifeStyles High Protein Dry Powder Shake plus 1 cup berries *(NO peanut butter)*	260	0

DINNER	CALORIES	FAT (g)
4 ounces very lean/lean protein OR 3 ounces very lean or lean protein plus 1 ounce cheese	140-220	0-12
1 heart-healthy fat servings *(add to very lean protein only)*	45	5
3 or more servings nonstarchy vegetables	45	0
½ cup fruit OR 1 cup berries	60-80	0

A dinner shake is no longer needed with the dinner meal, because introduction of fruit provides more carbohydrate options.

SAMPLE MENU

DAY 1

BREAKFAST:

- 20/20 LifeStyles High Protein Dry Powder Shake

- 1 tablespoon peanut butter

- ½ cup cut-up melon

LUNCH:

- 4 ounces tuna mixed with:

  ~ 1 tablespoon low-fat mayo

  ~ ½ cup diced celery (mix with tuna if desired)

  ~ 1 cup carrots

- 1 tennis-ball-sized orange

SNACK:

- 20/20 LifeStyles Protein Bar

DINNER:

- 4 ounces chicken breast, baked with 1 teaspoon oil

- 1½ cups steamed broccoli

- ¼ cup pineapple

- ½ cup strawberries

DAY 2

BREAKFAST:

- ½ cup low-fat cottage cheese mixed with:

  ~ ¼ cup peaches

  ~ ½ cup blueberries

  ~ 10 walnut halves

LUNCH:

- 4 ounces baked or grilled salmon

- Vegetable medley, steamed, including:

  ~ ½ cup cauliflower

  ~ ½ cup broccoli

  ~ ½ cup carrots

- 1 tennis-ball-sized apple

SNACK:

- 20/20 LifeStyles Protein Bar

DINNER:

- 4 ounces baked chicken breast

- Make a salad with:

  ~ 1½ cup spinach

  ~ ¼ cup radish

  ~ ¼ cup tomatoes

  ~ 1-2 tablespoons low-fat dressing

- ½ cup grapes

DAY 3

BREAKFAST:

- Scramble 1 cup Egg Beaters with 1 teaspoon oil

- 4 tablespoons salsa as a garnish

- ⅛ avocado

- 1 tennis-ball-sized apple

LUNCH:

- 4 ounces grilled beef tenderloin seasoned with pepper to taste

- 1½ cups steamed green beans

- 1 tennis-ball-sized plum

SNACK:

- 2 low-fat cheese sticks

- ½ cup clementine oranges

DINNER:

- 4 ounces turkey breast

- 6 almonds

- 1 cup steamed carrots

- ½ cup cooked spinach

- ½ cup pineapple

STAGE 4

Men 1,300-1,700 calories

BREAKFAST	CALORIES	FAT (g)
4 ounces very lean protein	140	0-4
2 heart-healthy fat servings *(see list for options)*	90	10
½ cup fruit OR 1 cup berries	60-80	0
OR		
Breakfast Shake Alternatives		

LUNCH	CALORIES	FAT (g)
6 ounces very lean/lean protein OR 5 ounces very lean or lean protein plus 1 ounce cheese	210-330	0-18
1 heart-healthy fat servings *(add to very lean protein only)*	45	5
3 or more servings nonstarchy vegetables	45	0
Choose one of the following		
1 cup berries OR ½ cup fruit	60-80	0

SNACK *(2 per day between lunch and dinner):* *Choose ONE of these options for your snack.*	CALORIES	FAT (g)
½ cup nonfat or low-fat cottage cheese plus ½ cup fruit	160-180	0-2
1 cup nonfat or low-fat plain Greek yogurt plus ½ cup fruit	140-170	0-4
2 ounces very lean protein plus 1 cup berries	130	0-2
20/20 LifeStyles High Protein Dry Powder Shake plus 1 cup berries *(NO peanut butter)*	260	0

DINNER	CALORIES	FAT (g)
6 ounces very lean/lean protein OR 5 ounces very lean or lean protein plus 1 ounce cheese	210-330	0-18
1 heart-healthy fat servings *(add to very lean protein only)*	45	5
3 or more servings nonstarchy vegetables	45	0
½ cup fruit OR 1 cup berries	60-80	0

A dinner shake is no longer needed with the dinner meal, because introduction of fruit provides more carbohydrate options.

SAMPLE MENU

DAY 1

BREAKFAST:

- 20/20 LifeStyles High Protein Dry Powder Shake

- 1 tablespoon peanut butter

- ½ cup peaches

SNACK:

- 2 sticks light string cheese

- 1 cup strawberries

LUNCH:

- 6 ounces tuna mixed with:

    - 1 tablespoon low-fat mayo

    - ½ cup diced celery (mix in with tuna if desired)

    - 1 cup carrots

- 1 tennis-ball-sized orange

SNACK:

- 20/20 LifeStyles Protein Bar

DINNER:

- 6 ounces chicken breast, cooked with 1 teaspoon oil

- 1½ cups steamed broccoli

- ½ cup cut-up honeydew melon

DAY 2

BREAKFAST:

- ½ cup low-fat cottage cheese mixed with:

    ~ ½ cup raspberries

    ~ ½ cup blueberries

    ~ 10 walnut halves

SNACK:

- 20/20 LifeStyles Protein Bar

LUNCH:

- 6 ounces salmon

- Vegetable medley, steamed, including:

    ~ ½ cup cauliflower

    ~ ½ cup broccoli

    ~ ½ cup carrots

- 1 tennis-ball-sized apple

SNACK:

2 ounces turkey breast

½ cup peaches

DINNER:

- 6 ounces chicken breast

- Make a salad with:

- 1½ cups spinach

- ½ cup radish

- ½ cup tomatoes

- 1-2 tablespoons low-fat dressing

- ½ cup grapes

DAY 3

BREAKFAST:

- Scramble 1 cup Egg Beaters in 1 teaspoon oil

- 4 tablespoons salsa as a garnish

- ⅛ avocado

- ½ cup melon

SNACK:

1 ounce low-sodium turkey jerky

1 tennis-ball-sized apple

LUNCH:

- 6 ounces grilled beef tenderloin, pepper to taste

- 1½ cups steamed green beans

- 1 tennis-ball-sized plum

SNACK:

- 2 low-fat cheese sticks

- ½ cup clementine oranges

DINNER:

- 6 ounces turkey

- 6 almonds

- 1 cup steamed carrots

- ½ cup cooked spinach

- ½ cup cut-up honeydew melon

EXERCISE PLAN:
AM I REALLY DOING THIS?

You're at the point now where you're just beginning to recognize your potential with exercise. You're starting to push aside the self-imposed mental barriers and do things you thought were impossible. The best competition you will ever win is the one you win against yourself, by surpassing those self-imposed limits. Enjoy!

Exercise Will Be As Follows

Level 1: Low fitness- Begin running with each workout if you can. High-speed walking for 40 minutes and running for 5 minutes at least five days per week. If running is difficult for you, add an additional 5 minutes of high-speed walking. You may have to walk up a gradual hill to keep your heart rate high. Keep your pace at a level to reach your optimum heart rate range (65-85 percent of your maximum).

Level 2: Moderate fitness- We will start doing interval training. That means you alternate high-intensity and moderate-intensity exercise. Start with high-speed walking for 10 minutes, then running or hill-walking for 10 minutes; next, a second set of high-speed walking for 10 minutes, then running or hill-walking for 15 minutes. Do this at least five days per week. You should keep your heart rate at optimum level (65-85 percent of your maximum).

Level 3: High fitness- Running for 45 minutes at least five days per week. Continue running gradual hills and keeping your heart rate at optimum level. Start timing your runs. Work toward being able to run 6 miles in 60 minutes, or faster if you can.

All Levels: Keep wearing your pedometers and keep your steps at or above 6,000 per day, excluding exercise.

Now is the time to start exploring active sports that seem like they would be enjoyable for you-such activities as racquetball, squash, skiing, hiking, bicycling, etc. Take a lesson in one of these activities. You don't have to be perfect; the goal is to find something active you enjoy. If you're a family person, try to find something the whole family can do. You may want to join a health club and try a number of different activities. As long as you can keep your heart rate at optimum level (65-85 percent of your maximum), feel free to trade off some of your walking and running days for an activity like hiking, cycling, spinning, TRX, or CrossFit, but be sure to keep your heart rate continuously at the optimum level.

LIFESTYLE PLAN:
WHY DO I DO THESE THINGS?

Habits are difficult to form, but they're even harder to change or eliminate. There's a reason for that: Habits are very useful to us. Imagine driving down the road and thinking of moving your right foot to the brake, then thinking how hard to press and when to start pressing every time you had to stop. It would be like learning to drive every time you got into your car. Habits make this unnecessary. You see the stop sign, and you automatically stop-no thought involved. You do this many thousands of times per day in many routine situations. You save your brain power for novel or creative tasks. Without this ability to form habits, human beings would be very inefficient and could not have evolved to our current level.

Unfortunately, though, some habits are not so useful. Eating chips while watching TV, drinking beer at the game, stopping at the Starbucks on the way home for a double Frappuccino or stopping at Cinnabon in the mall.

Most of what we call "mindless" eating is a habit and actually is almost mindless.

Habits are stored at the base of your brain in the basal ganglia. The basal ganglia are located almost as far down in the brainstem as the autonomic areas that control such things as your heartbeat and your breathing. Because these functions require little thought, they're called autonomic, which means automatic.

Habits are created by repetition of behaviors. Once created, they tend to be automatic. The habit cycle begins with a cue. A cue alerts your brain that a set of stored behaviors in your brain is required to deal with something in your environment. An example might be walking through the mall and smelling the bakery. The bakery smell is the cue. When a habit responds to a cue, we say the habit is being cued. If you have smelled this smell on many occasions and responded to the smell by buying and eating a pastry, you've created a habit.

So, smelling the pastry cues your habit, and the result is that you almost automatically buy and eat the pastry. You do this without conscious thought.

Many different types of environmental stimuli can cue you. Your senses of smell, taste, sight, or sound can cue you; so can time of day, holidays, locations, people, or emotions.

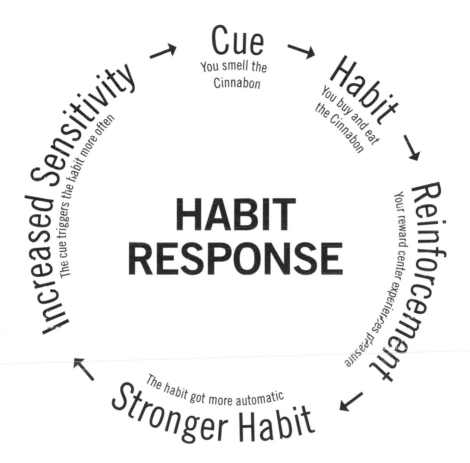

One way to deal with these habits is to remove the cues from your environment. Don't drive home past your favorite Frappuccino store. Get the junk food out of the house.

Don't eat at the restaurant where you normally overeat.

You must identify your unhealthy habits and the cues that trigger them. Habits can be difficult to identify, because they're so much a part of you that you don't notice them. In order to discover your habits, take 15 minutes today and start writing down the unhealthy habits you had before you started our food plan. If that's difficult, enlist the aid of your support person, a close friend, or a family member. Now you have a list of the habits that need changing. Keep this list on your smartphone or computer, because they will help remind you of other habits that need to be changed.

The most powerful habit that exists is the keystone habit(30). Many of you know that the keystone was the center stone on a Roman arch that kept the arch suspended. The Roman arch was the wonder of the world for more than a millennium. And, like the stone that supports the arch, each of you also has keystone habits that support groups of other habits. Change the keystone habits and the others change automatically.

Here's an example. Suppose you actually eat very little during the day, but from the end of a late dinner at 8:00 p.m. until you go to bed at 1:00 a.m., you eat nonstop. A keystone habit would be your sleep schedule. If you alter your sleep time, going to bed at 9:30 p.m., the night binging habit collapses.

Another example is snacking while watching TV. The keystone habit here is watching TV. Find more active entertainment, or only watch TV with a group of "normal" eaters and the habit collapses.

Now, look at your habit list and see if you can identify the keystone habits that lead to the destructive habits that have caused your weight gain. Develop a plan to modify those habits, then, get your support people to assist you in making those changes. Expect that those habits will, however, take a considerable time to fully change.

---

30. Charles Duhigg, *The Power of Habit: Why We Do What We Do In Life and Business,* Random House, 2012.

We have repeatedly seen how our patients gained weight as a result of unhealthy eating and lifestyle habits, and we've helped them change these habits. Use the techniques we discussed above to take control of your unhealthy eating habits.

Much more information on changing habits is available in videos Reward Center 3-5 under Nutrition at www.2020lifestyles.com/resources-tools/educational-videos.aspx

Discovering and modifying habits can be difficult. If you need help changing these destructive patterns and you live in the Puget Sound area, contact one of our counselors at:
www.prohub.com/Wellness/Counseling

CHAPTER 12

PUTTING IT ALL TOGETHER

STAGE 5, STAGE 6 AND STAGE 7

Stage 5 introduces all dairy products back into the meal plan, including regular yogurt and milk. In this stage, when we refer to dairy, we include fruit-flavored yogurts as well as low-fat cheese, Greek yogurt, and nonfat and low-fat milk. Now, 1 serving of dairy is equivalent to 1 cup of nonfat or low-fat milk or ½ cup fruit- flavored yogurt. To make sure you don't slow down your weight loss, continue to limit your total intake of dairy products to 0-2 servings per day. If you find dairy does slow or stop your weight loss, remove dairy from your plan, because it's not necessary.

In Stage 3, skim milk and 1 percent milk were classed as high-protein items, however, regular and fruit-flavored (non-Greek) yogurts are considered a carbohydrate. Yogurts that are not labeled as "Greek" are low in protein, and their carbohydrate content makes up from 2-3 times their protein content. Also, remember that in Stage 4 we pointed out the advantage of pairing all carbohydrates with a protein or a healthy fat. This same rule now applies to milk and regular yogurts. For a snack, pair a carbohydrate-based dairy item with a protein, such as ¼ cup cottage cheese, 2 ounces of grilled chicken strips, or 2 ounces of low-sodium deli ham slices. Keep in mind that your deli meats should contain less than 500 mg sodium per serving, and if you have high blood pressure, you must avoid them altogether.

Here are some guidelines to help you when choosing a regular, non-Greek yogurt: Read the label and aim for these guidelines per ½ cup serving:

> *Less than or equal to 130 calories per serving*

> *And less than or equal to 16 grams of sugar*

Following these rules will help avoid excess sugar.

At this time you may introduce fruit-flavored Greek yogurts. Since the protein to carbohydrate ratio in the food is approximately 1:1, think of these items as having a built-in protein with the carbohydrate already found in the yogurt. Flavored Greek yogurts are perfect when you're on the run, because they're a balanced snack, and all in one portable container.

> *Greek or high-protein yogurt is considered a protein (Stage 3). These yogurts have more protein than carbohydrates.*

> *Other fruit-flavored yogurts that are NOT Greek are considered a carbohydrate (Stage 5), because the protein is half of the total carbohydrates.*

> *Fruit-flavored Greek yogurts have both protein and added carbohydrates. When the protein and carbohydrates are in a 1:1 ratio (almost equal in gram amounts), we consider this a hybrid! Basically, it is BOTH a protein, and a carbohydrate (Stage 5). Make sure to read labels to see what category your yogurt choice falls into!*

For lunch and dinner, your meal will consist of protein, vegetables, heart-healthy fat if needed, and one carbohydrate serving. Now, you have multiple carbohydrate options to choose from for your meals: 1 cup berries, or ½ cup fruit, or 1 cup milk, or ½ cup non-Greek yogurt.

As we said before, dairy products have been known to slow down weight loss. Your body gets all the nutrients it needs from protein, vegetables, and berries. Dairy products are not a required part of your meal plan. Good luck with Stage 5 this week.

STAGE 5

MEAL PLAN: DAIRY DELIGHT

Stage 5 includes low-fat milk, skim milk, fruit-flavored yogurt, and fruit-flavored Greek yogurt.

Servings: 0-2 servings of all dairy-based products per day for men and women

Serving Sizes:

- 1 percent reduced-fat or skim milk: 1 serving = 1 cup*

- Fruit-flavored (non-Greek) yogurt: 1 serving = ½ cup*

Nonfat and low-fat milk are also included in Stage 5. These items are carbohydrates and need to be paired with a protein or healthy fat.

- Fruit-flavored Greek yogurt: 1 serving = ½ cup

Fruit-flavored Greek yogurts (hybrid yogurts) are balanced. They have BOTH carbohydrates and protein.

Calorie range: 60-120 calories per serving

SHOPPING LIST: YOGURT

Higher-Carbohydrate Yogurts

These yogurts meet the criterion of 25 grams carbohydrate maximum per 7 grams of protein. For snacks, remember to pair a protein or a healthy fat with these yogurts.

- ☐ Yami, Wallaby, Stony Field brands
- ☐ Rachel's
- ☐ All Plain Nonfat and Low Fat yogurts meet these guidelines.

Hybrid Yogurts

These yogurts are high-protein yogurts with fruit or sweetener and have close to a 1:1 carbohydrate to protein ratio. These can be enjoyed alone as a snack.

- ☐ Trader Joe's 0 percent flavored Greek yogurt
- ☐ Voskos 0 percent flavored Greek yogurt
- ☐ Oikos 0 percent flavored Greek yogurt
- ☐ Chobani 0 percent Greek yogurt
- ☐ Siggi's Icelandic 0 percent flavored Greek yogurt

STAGE 5

Women 1,100-1,400 calories

BREAKFAST	CALORIES	FAT (g)
4 ounces very lean protein	140	0-4
2 heart-healthy fat servings *(see list for options)*	90	10
1 cup berries OR ½ cup fruit	60-80	0
OR		
Breakfast Shake Alternatives		

LUNCH	CALORIES	FAT (g)
4 ounces very lean/lean protein OR 3 ounces very lean or lean protein plus 1 ounce cheese	140-220	0-12
1 heart-healthy fat servings *(add to very lean protein only)*	45	5
3 or more servings nonstarchy vegetables	45	0
Choose ONE of the carbohydrate choices listed below:		
1 cup berries, ½ cup fruit, ½ cup nonfat or low-fat flavored yogurt OR 1 cup nonfat or low-fat milk	60-100	0-3

SNACK *(1 per day between lunch and dinner)*	CALORIES	FAT (g)
½ cup nonfat flavored Greek yogurt plus 1-2 tablespoons nuts or seeds	140-220	5-10
¼ cup nonfat or low-fat cottage cheese plus ½ cup nonfat or low-fat flavored yogurt	190-220	0-4
2 ounces very lean protein plus 1 cup berries	130	0-2
20/20 LifeStyles High Protein Dry Powder Shake plus 1 cup berries *(NO peanut butter)*	260	0

DINNER	CALORIES	FAT (g)
4 ounces very lean/lean protein OR 3 ounces very lean or lean protein plus 1 ounce cheese	140-220	0-12
1 heart-healthy fat servings *(add to very lean protein only)*	45	5
3 or more servings nonstarchy vegetables	45	0
Choose ONE of the carbohydrate choices listed below:		
1 cup berries, ½ cup fruit, ½ cup nonfat or low-fat flavored yogurt, and 1 cup nonfat or low-fat milk	60-100	0-3

SAMPLE MENU

DAY 1

BREAKFAST:

- 20/20 LifeStyles High Protein Dry Powder Shake

- 1 tablespoon peanut butter

- 1 cup blueberries

LUNCH:

- 4 ounces pork tenderloin

- 1½ cups broccoli

- 1 tennis-ball-sized apple

SNACK:

- 20/20 LifeStyles Protein Bar

DINNER:

- 25 large shrimp

- 2 teaspoons cooking oil

- 1½ cups asparagus

- ½ cup nonfat blueberry flavored yogurt

DAY 2

BREAKFAST:

- 1 cup low-fat strawberry flavored yogurt

- 2 whole eggs plus 2 egg whites scrambled

LUNCH:

- 4 ounces chicken breast
- Make a salad with:
    ~ 1½ cups spinach
    ~ ¼ cup tomato
    ~ ¼ cup mushroom
    ~ ½ cup carrots
    ~ ⅛ avocado
    ~ 2-4 tablespoons salsa as a garnish
- 1 tennis-ball-sized peach

SNACK:

- 2 ounces low-sodium deli ham
- ½ cup melon

DINNER:

- Lettuce wrap burger made with :
    ~ 4 ounces very lean ground beef (4-5 percent fat) patty
    ~ ⅛ avocado
    ~ Mustard
    ~ 1 tablespoon ketchup
    ~ 1 tomato slice
    ~ 1-2 large lettuce leaves as the wrap
- 1 cup carrots
- 1 cup nonfat milk

DAY 3

BREAKFAST:

- Using 1 teaspoon oil, scramble:
    - ~ 6 egg whites
    - ~ 1 ounce chicken sausage
    - ~ 1 tablespoon peanut butter
- 1 tennis-ball-sized apple

LUNCH:

- Tuna wrap made with:
    - ~ 4 ounces canned tuna
    - ~ 1 tablespoon low-fat mayo
    - ~ 1-2 lettuce leaves for wrap (optional)
- 1 cup green beans
- 1 tennis-ball-sized peach

SNACK:

- 6 ounces flavored nonfat Greek yogurt plus 1-2 tablespoons nuts or seeds

DINNER:

- 4 ounces baked salmon
- 1½ cups steamed broccoli
- 1 cup mixed berries

STAGE 5

Men 1,300-1,700 calories

BREAKFAST	CALORIES	FAT (g)
4 ounces very lean protein	140	0-4
2 heart-healthy fat servings *(see list for options)*	90	10
1 cup berries OR ½ cup fruit	60-80	0
OR		
Breakfast Shake Alternatives		

LUNCH	CALORIES	FAT (g)
6 ounces very lean/lean protein OR 5 ounces very lean or lean protein plus 1 ounce cheese	210-330	0-18
1 heart-healthy fat servings *(add to very lean protein only)*	45	5
3 or more servings nonstarchy vegetables	45	0
Choose ONE of the carbohydrate choices listed below:		
1 cup berries, ½ cup fruit, ½ cup nonfat or low-fat flavored yogurt OR 1 cup nonfat or low-fat milk	60-100	0-3

SNACK *(2 per day between lunch and dinner)*: *Choose ONE of these options for your snack.*	CALORIES	FAT (g)
½ cup nonfat flavored Greek yogurt plus 1-2 tablespoons nuts or seeds	140-220	5-10
¼ cup nonfat or low-fat cottage cheese plus ½ cup nonfat or low-fat flavored yogurt	190-220	0-4
2 ounces very lean protein plus 1 cup berries	130	0-2
20/20 LifeStyles High Protein Dry Powder Shake plus 1 cup berries *(NO peanut butter)*	260	0

DINNER	CALORIES	FAT (g)
6 ounces very lean/lean protein OR 5 ounces very lean or lean protein plus 1 ounce cheese	210-330	0-18
1 heart-healthy fat servings *(add to very lean protein only)*	45	5
3 or more servings nonstarchy vegetables	45	0
Choose ONE of the carbohydrate choices listed below:		
1 cup berries, ½ cup fruit, ½ cup nonfat or low-fat flavored yogurt, and 1 cup nonfat or low-fat milk	60-100	0-3

SAMPLE MENU

DAY 1

BREAKFAST:

- 20/20 LifeStyles High Protein Dry Powder Shake

- 1 tablespoon peanut butter

- ½ cup mixed fruit

SNACK:

- 20/20 LifeStyles Protein Bar

LUNCH:

- 6 ounces baked pork tenderloin

- 1½ cups broccoli

- 1 tennis-ball-sized apple

SNACK:

- 2 ounces low-sodium deli ham

- ½ cup melon

DINNER:

- In 2 teaspoons cooking oil, sauté:

    ~ 25 large shrimp

    ~ 1½ cups asparagus

- 1 cup low-fat peach-flavored yogurt

DAY 2

BREAKFAST:

- 1 cup nonfat strawberry-flavored yogurt
- 2 whole eggs plus 2 egg whites scrambled

SNACK:

- 1 tennis-ball-sized apple
- 1 tablespoon peanut butter

LUNCH:

- 6 ounces chicken breast
- Make a salad with:
    - 1½ cups spinach
    - ¼ cup tomato
    - ¼ cup mushroom
    - ½ cup carrots
    - ⅛ avocado
    - 2-4 tablespoons salsa as garnish
- 1 tennis-ball-sized peach

SNACK:

- ½ cup shelled edamame
- 1 tennis-ball-sized orange

DINNER:

- Lettuce wrap burger made with:
    - ~ 6 ounces very lean ground beef (4-5 percent fat) patty
    - ~ ⅛ avocado
    - ~ Mustard
    - ~ 1 tablespoon ketchup
    - ~ 1 tomato slice
    - ~ 1-2 large lettuce leaves as wrap
- 1 cup carrots
- 1 cup nonfat milk

DAY 3

BREAKFAST:

- Using 1 teaspoon oil, scramble:
    - ~ 6 egg whites
    - ~ 1 ounce chicken or ham
- 1 tablespoon peanut butter
- 1 tennis-ball-sized apple

SNACK:

- 2 ounces grilled chicken breast
- 1 cup strawberries

LUNCH:

- Tuna salad or wrap made with:

    ~ 6 ounces tuna

    ~ 1 tablespoon low-fat mayo

    ~ 1-2 lettuce leaves for wrap (optional)

- 1 cup sugar snap peas

- ½ cup nonfat pineapple-flavored yogurt

SNACK:

- ½ cup Greek yogurt plus 1-2 tablespoons nuts or seeds

DINNER:

- 6 ounces baked salmon

- 1½ cups steamed broccoli

- 1 cup mixed berries

EXERCISE PLAN: LOOK AT ME!

You used to see the really fit people as a separate group that was very different from yourself. Now, you're starting to see that you can be like them. In fact, following the guidelines in this book will make you one of them. So let's push on. You're doing great, but you still have a long, exciting way to go, to realize your potential.

Exercise Will Be As Follows:

Level 1: Low fitness- High-speed walking for 10 minutes and running or hill walking for 5 minutes. Repeat this three times in a row to accumulate 45 minutes of exercise, at least five days per week. Keep your pace at a level to reach your optimum heart rate range (65-85 percent of your maximum).

Level 2: Moderate fitness- High-speed walking for 12 minutes, then running or hill walking for 20 minutes, and finally high-speed walking for 12 minutes, at least five days per week. You should keep your heart rate at optimum level (65-85 percent of your maximum).

Level 3: High fitness- Running for 45 minutes at least five days per week. Continue running gradual hills. Heart rate at optimum level. Continue timing your runs. Continue working up to 6 miles in 60 minutes or better (no change from Stage 4 yet).

All Levels: Keep wearing your pedometers and keep your steps at 6,000 per day, excluding exercise. Keep exploring active sports for yourself and your friends or family.

LIFESTYLE PLAN: THE TRUTH TABLET

Somehow writing things down helps us to see things more clearly. In Concept #18, we talked about your thoughts passing the truth test. Writing things down helps you do that, and that's important, but it also helps you do much more.

Writing can help you make difficult decisions. Write the decision you must make at the top of the page and then, in two columns beneath that, write the heading: Advantages-Disadvantages.

Now, list all the advantages and disadvantages of all the various choices you might make. Talk this over with your support person, a family member, friend, or trusted advisor. You will find that this takes a lot of the guesswork and a lot of the stress out of decision-making.

Here Is a Decision Log example:

JOB OFFER FROM NEW COMPANY			
Take offer		**Stay at current job**	
Advantage	Disadvantage	Advantage	Disadvantage
More money	Have to prove myself again	Respected here	Less money
Manager position	Don't know staff	May be manager soon	Unsure of promotion
A new challenge	New stresses	Little stress	A bit bored at work
	Have to move	Like my city/house	
	Kids change school	Kids like current school	
	Wife likes her job	Keep wife happy	

It becomes fairly obvious that your new job's disadvantages seem to outweigh the advantages, and your decision gets much easier.

You can also track your life by keeping a mood log. Keep track of the following moods:

- Anger/irritability

- Depression/moodiness

- Anxiety/stress.

Use the scale of 0 equals none of that feeling to 10 equals the worst it's ever been. Now, down the left side of the page write the date, day, and time. Next to that, write a very short description of what's currently happening. Do this at least 6-10 times a day.

Here Is a Mood Log example:

	Anger	Depression	Anxiety
Tue, Jan 3, 9:00 a.m. *Annual review with boss*	3	3	6
Tue, Jan 3, 12:00 p.m. *Lunch with co-worker*	1	1	1
Tue, Jan 3, 6:00 p.m. *On way home*	0	5	5
Tue, Jan 3, 8:00 p.m. *Difficulty getting kids to bed*	5	5	5

Analyzing this log, we can see several things. Your job causes significant stress in your life. Also, parenting is an issue that needs some attention, since it causes a number of unpleasant feelings. Remember that stress and depression cause the body to produce cortisol, and cortisol makes you hungry.

Now that you've identified the issues, you can begin to resolve them. Talk to your family and support group. If you still have unresolved issues, talk to a psychologist or counselor in your area. If you live in the Puget Sound area, talk to one of our psychologists or counselors at: https://www.proclub.com/Wellness/Counseling

The Mood Log is a valuable tool to get some answers about your life, and why you feel and behave the way you do. Examining your logs for patterns will give you great insight into what's affecting you, and what you have to do about it.

STAGE 6

In Stage 6, we introduce legumes. This includes beans, lentils, and split peas. Beans, the most commonly consumed food in the legume family, contain a small amount of protein. But as beans actually have 2-3 times more carbohydrate content than protein, they must be considered a carbohydrate. One serving of beans is equal to ½ cup, which is equal to 100 calories. You can start by adding 1-2 servings of beans per day if you'd like, but only ONE per meal. Remember to measure your carbohydrates accurately and limit them to one carbohydrate serving per meal. Only use carbohydrate options you enjoy. If you aren't a fan of beans, or if your hunger returns, feel free to follow the Stage 5 plan for another week or longer.

Again, ½ cup of cooked beans has 100 calories. Remember the last time you went out for Mexican food? How many servings of beans were on your plate? Probably 2-3 on the side of your main dish. Remember, ½ cup equals 100 calories, so 2-3 servings equals 200 to 300 calories, not including the entree. The burrito has another 800 calories, and if we add another 100 for the sour cream on top, 200 for the guacamole, 300 or more for a side of rice, and another 200 for the cheese drenching the burrito, rice, and beans. And this doesn't even include the basket of chips you ate before the meal (up to 500 calories) **for a grand total of 2,400 calories**. Many restaurant meals are very high in calories, and not just in Mexican restaurants. Always be mindful of portion size and the calorie content of your food when you are dining out. As you may have noticed, all food groups introduced from Stage 4 on, are a carbohydrate choice. Here's where things get tricky.

You should only choose ONE carbohydrate food at each meal and snack to keep calories within plan, keep your blood sugar level, and keep all meals and snacks appropriately balanced.

As we introduce beans in Stage 6, it opens up the world of hummus. Hummus is another "hybrid" food, in that it has a built-in healthy fat paired with the carbohydrate. Hummus is made from puréed garbanzo beans, tahini or sesame paste, and extra virgin olive oil. It should be treated as a carbohydrate, but since the hummus has fat already in it, pairing it with a protein is optional. Consume a maximum of 2-4 level, not heaping tablespoons per serving. This means that hummus is a balanced snack all on its own. A snack idea is 2 ounces sliced lean turkey or raw sliced bell peppers with 2 tablespoons of hummus, a Mediterranean treat in mid-afternoon to tide you over until dinner, and it's only 110 calories, 12 grams of protein, 6 grams of carbohydrates, and 4 grams of fat. **It is essential that you carefully measure your portions of hummus, because it's easy to consume too much.**

Follow these guidelines when choosing canned beans:

Low-sodium beans: Include only beans with less than 400 mg of sodium per ½ cup serving.

Rinse beans for 1 minute to decrease the sodium content by nearly 25 percent. Also, buy no salt added or low-sodium beans when you can. Cooking beans from their dry form in a pressure cooker, although time consuming, can help you to avoid excess sodium.

Be sure to see the chili recipes in appendix H. To increase the protein content of the chili, use high-protein nonfat Greek yogurt as a sour-cream substitute. Top your chili with ⅛ avocado for a tasty, healthy-fat serving.

You will notice that there are no soups in this plan. That's because soup, like fruit juice, is liquid calories, and liquid calories give no satiety unless they contain at least 20 grams of protein. Remember, for carbohydrates, ONE serving per meal, and keep measuring and tracking your foods!

From this point on we'll be guiding you into the "new normal." We're fine-tuning your nutritional plan in a way that will keep you at a normal weight and healthy for life. Continue to be diligent with your meal tracking, as this tool becomes even more important as we add back food groups. Remember to keep your water intake up as well. Good luck with Stage 6!

MEAL PLAN: CHILI TIME

Stage 6 includes Beans (all varieties), lentils, split peas (these items are carbohydrates)

Servings: 0-2 servings per day for men and women

Serving sizes:

-1 serving = ½ cup cooked

Calories: ½ cup = 100 calories

SHOPPING LIST: LEGUMES

Low-sodium canned beans: Eden Organic, Westbrae Natural, Progresso, S&W 50 percent Less Salt.

Refried beans: Rosarita No Fat Traditional Refried Beans (sodium 520 mg per ½ cup)

Serving Suggestions

Beans absorb the flavors of foods they are cooked with. Try these seasoning ideas:	
Mexican	Hot peppers, garlic, cilantro
Italian	Garlic, oregano, basil, sage, rosemary
Indian	Curry, turmeric, cumin, coriander, cayenne, ginger

- *Make a bean salad or add beans to salad greens.*

  - Mix black beans or nonfat refried beans with salsa for a side dish.

- *Beans can make tasty spreads and dips.*

  - Hummus can be a great snack, especially when paired with nonstarchy vegetables or hardboiled egg whites. (Note: 2-4 tablespoons can be a snack-size portion for hummus. As 4 tablespoons of hummus yield 100 calories, do not exceed this serving size.)

STAGE 6

Women 1,100-1,400 calories

BREAKFAST	CALORIES	FAT (g)
4 ounces very lean protein	140	0-4
2 heart-healthy fat servings *(see list for options)*	90	10
1 cup berries OR ½ cup fruit	60-80	0
OR		
Breakfast Shake Alternatives		

LUNCH	CALORIES	FAT (g)
4 ounces very lean/lean protein OR 3 ounces very lean or lean protein plus 1 ounce cheese	140-220	0-12
1 heart-healthy fat servings *(add to very lean protein only)*	45	5
3 or more servings nonstarchy vegetables	45	0
Choose ONE of the carbohydrate choices listed below:		
1 cup berries, ½ cup fruit, ½ cup nonfat or low-fat flavored yogurt, 1 cup nonfat or low-fat milk OR ½ cup cooked beans	60-100	0-3

SNACK *(1 per day between lunch and dinner)*	CALORIES	FAT (g)
Halve 2 hardboiled eggs, discard the yolks, and stuff with 4 tablespoons hummus	135	4-6
¼ cup hummus plus ½ cup mixed vegetables	130	4-6
2 ounces very lean protein plus 1 cup berries	130	0-2
20/20 LifeStyles High Protein Dry Powder Shake plus 1 cup berries *(NO peanut butter)*	260	0

DINNER	CALORIES	FAT (g)
4 ounces very lean/lean protein OR 3 ounces very lean or lean protein plus 1 ounce cheese	140-220	0-12
1 heart-healthy fat servings *(add to very lean protein only)*	45	5
3 or more servings nonstarchy vegetables	45	0
Choose ONE of the carbohydrate choices listed below:		
1 cup berries, ½ cup fruit, ½ cup nonfat or low-fat flavored yogurt, 1 cup nonfat or low-fat milk OR ½ cup cooked beans	60-100	0-3

SAMPLE MENU

DAY 1

BREAKFAST:

- 20/20 LifeStyles High Protein Dry Powder Shake

- 1 tablespoon almond butter

- ½ cup mango

LUNCH:

- 4 ounces chicken breast, baked with 1 teaspoon oil

- 1 cup steamed cauliflower

- ½ cup steamed carrots

- 1-2 teaspoons freshly grated Parmesan cheese as garnish

- 1 cup strawberries

SNACK:

- 20/20 LifeStyles Protein Bar

DINNER:

- 4 ounces grilled pork tenderloin

- ½ cup low-sodium pinto beans

- Make a salad with:

  - 1½ cups romaine lettuce

  - ½ cup tomatoes

  - ½ cup sliced cucumber

  - Fresh salsa as garnish

DAY 2

BREAKFAST:

- Scramble:
    - ~ 6 egg whites
    - ~ 1 ounce ham
- 12 almonds
- ½ cup blueberries
- 4 ounces nonfat milk

LUNCH:

- 4 ounces baked cod
- Make a salad with:
    - ~ 1½ cup arugula
    - ~ 1 cup mixed vegetables *(tomatoes, carrots, celery, mushrooms, etc.)*
    - ~ 2 tablespoons low-fat salad dressing
- 1 cup raspberries

SNACK:

- 1 low-fat cheese stick
- 1 ounce low-sodium deli turkey
- 1 tennis-ball-sized apple

DINNER:

- 4 ounces baked lamb, trimmed of visible fat
- ½ cup steamed carrots

- 1 cup steamed asparagus

- ½ cup mixed tropical fruit

DAY 3

BREAKFAST:

- Mix:

- ½ cup nonfat plain Greek yogurt

- ½ cup nonfat blueberry flavored yogurt

- 10 walnut halves

LUNCH:

- 4 ounces chicken breast

- Make a salad with:

    ~ ½ cup garbanzo beans

    ~ 1½ cups spinach

    ~ ½ cup tomatoes

    ~ ½ cup carrots

    ~ 1-2 tablespoons low-fat dressing

SNACK:

- Halve 2 hardboiled eggs, remove yolks, and stuff whites
  with 4 tablespoons hummus

DINNER:

- 4 ounces baked rib roast, trimmed of visible fat

- 1½ cups steamed broccoli

- 1 small apple

STAGE 6

Men 1,300-1,700 calories

BREAKFAST	CALORIES	FAT (g)
4 ounces very lean protein	140	0-4
2 heart-healthy fat servings *(see list for options)*	90	10
1 cup berries OR ½ cup fruit	60-80	0
OR		
Breakfast Shake Alternatives		

LUNCH	CALORIES	FAT (g)
6 ounces very lean/lean protein OR 5 ounces very lean or lean protein plus 1 ounce cheese	210-330	0-18
1 heart-healthy fat servings *(add to very lean protein only)*	45	5
3 or more servings nonstarchy vegetables	45	0
Choose ONE of the carbohydrate choices listed below:		
1 cup berries, ½ cup fruit, ½ cup nonfat or low-fat flavored yogurt, 1 cup nonfat or low-fat milk OR ½ cup cooked beans	60-100	0-3

SNACK *(2 per day between lunch and dinner)*: *Choose ONE of these options for your snack.*	CALORIES	FAT (g)
Halve 2 hardboiled eggs, remove yolks, and stuff whites with 4 tablespoons hummus	135	4-6
¼ cup hummus plus ½ cup mixed vegetables	130	4-6
2 ounces very lean protein plus 1 cup berries	130	0-2
20/20 LifeStyles High Protein Dry Powder Shake plus 1 cup berries *(NO peanut butter)*	260	0

DINNER	CALORIES	FAT (g)
6 ounces very lean/lean protein OR 5 ounces very lean or lean protein plus 1 ounce cheese	210-330	0-18
1 heart-healthy fat servings *(add to very lean protein only)*	45	5
3 or more servings nonstarchy vegetables	45	0
Choose ONE of the carbohydrate choices listed below:		
1 cup berries, ½ cup fruit, ½ cup nonfat or low-fat flavored yogurt, 1 cup nonfat or low-fat milk OR ½ cup cooked beans	60-100	0-3

SAMPLE MENU

DAY 1

BREAKFAST:

- 20/20 LifeStyles High Protein Dry Powder Shake

- 1 tablespoon peanut butter

- ½ cup pineapple

SNACK

- 2 tablespoons hummus

- 2 ounces chicken strips

- ½ cup carrots

LUNCH:

- 6 ounces chicken breast, baked with 1 teaspoon oil

- 1 cup steamed cauliflower

- ½ cup steamed carrots

- 1 cup strawberries

SNACK:

20/20 LifeStyles Protein Bar

DINNER:

- 6 ounces baked pork tenderloin

- ½ cup low-sodium pinto beans

- Make a salad with:

    ~ 1½ cup romaine lettuce

    ~ ½ cup tomatoes

    ~ ½ cup sliced cucumber

    ~ Fresh salsa as garnish

DAY 2

BREAKFAST:

- Scramble:

    ~ 6 egg whites

    ~ 1 ounce low-sodium ham

- 12 almonds

- 1 cup blueberries

- 1 tennis-ball-sized orange

SNACK:

- Halve 2 hardboiled eggs, remove yolks, and stuff whites with 4 tablespoons hummus

LUNCH:

- 6 ounces baked cod
- Make a salad with:
    - 1½ cup arugula
    - 1 cup mixed vegetables *(tomatoes, carrots, celery, mushrooms, etc.)*
    - 1-2 tablespoons low-fat salad dressing
- 1 cup raspberries

SNACK:

- 2 low-fat cheese sticks
- 1 apple

DINNER:

- 6 ounces baked lamb, trimmed of fat
- ½ cup steamed carrots
- 1 cup steamed asparagus
- ½ cup cubed mango

DAY 3

BREAKFAST:

- Mix:

    ~ ½ cup nonfat plain Greek yogurt

    ~ ½ cup blueberry-flavored yogurt

    ~ 10 walnut halves

SNACK:

- 2 ounces low-sodium deli ham

- ½ cup cantaloupe

LUNCH:

- 6 ounces chicken breast

- Make a salad with:

    ~ ½ cup garbanzo beans

    ~ 1½ cups spinach

    ~ ¼ cup chopped tomato

    ~ ¼ cup carrots

    ~ 1-2 tablespoons light dressing

SNACK:

- 3 tablespoons hummus

- ½ cup carrots

- 2 ounces grilled chicken breast

DINNER:

- 6 ounces baked rib roast, trimmed of fat

- 1½ cups steamed broccoli

- 1 tennis-ball-sized apple

EXERCISE PLAN: A NEW HABIT

Level 1: Low fitness- High-speed walking for 5 minutes and running or hill walking for 10 minutes. Repeat three times in a row to accumulate 45 minutes of exercise, at least 5 days per week. Keep your pace at a level to reach your optimum heart rate range (65-85 percent of your maximum).

Level 2: Moderate fitness- High-speed walking for 10 minutes and running or hill walking for 30 minutes and high-speed walking for 5 minutes, at least 5 days per week. Keep your heart rate at optimum level (65-85 percent of your maximum).

Level 3: High fitness- Running 6 miles, 4 days per week (5th day optional), and 8 miles once a week. Continue running gradual hills. Heart rate at optimum level. Continue timing your runs, working up to 6 miles in 48 minutes or better. Enter a 10K race in your area.

All Levels: Keep wearing your pedometer when not exercising, and keep your steps at 6,000 or more per day, excluding your exercise routine.

LIFESTYLE PLAN: MINDFUL EATING

One of the problems we've seen in many of our patients is that they eat in a manner that makes it impossible for them to reach satiety either physically or psychologically. This is mindless eating, characterized by eating so rapidly that your body and mind cannot register satiety, or by eating while doing other things that distract you from your awareness of eating. An example of the latter is snacking at a meeting or while watching TV. It takes 15-20 minutes for your body chemistry to communicate to your brain that you have eaten.

Mindful eating means that you will slow your eating and make it an event. You will focus on eating in order to give your body and your mind a chance to catch up and give you satiety. You will take a moment to see your food, slowly consume it by methodically chewing, tasting, and swallowing.

Here are the steps to accomplish mindful eating:

- Water belongs on the table; maybe with a slice of lemon, no matter where you're eating-at home or away. Always have water on the table.

- Look at your plate of food and appreciate what is in front of you. Take a moment to anticipate eating it.

- As you eat, remember this is a sensory experience. It's important to be aware of every bite and how it feels in your mouth, its aromas, and its flavors. Try to identify each spice used in the preparation of this meal. Take your time! Enjoy.

- Place your fork, spoon, or knife back on the plate between each bite. Before you pick up your fork, have a sip of water.

- Be the last one to finish eating. This will be a new experience for many of you.

- Time how long it takes you to eat. Timing your meal will help you eat more slowly. Research shows that when you eat more slowly, you consume fewer calories.

- Do not eat in front of the television set. Make eating a food-focused event.

- As always, be sure to meal track.

In Chapter 11, we talked about habits and cues. Mindful eating will remove many of the cues that have been triggering your mindless or habit eating.

STAGE 7
MEAL PLAN: THE DANGER ZONE

The last food group we introduce to your food plan is whole grains. These include everything from bread, rice, pasta, and cereal to such snack foods as pretzels and crackers. Because of their high starch content, we also include starchy vegetables in this group. Starchy vegetables, such as corn, peas, potatoes, sweet potatoes, and winter squash, are considered simple carbohydrates, but because they have a high calorie content, we group them with the whole-grain foods.

Remember that starch and sugar are synonymous. For your health, make up your mind to eat only whole-grain products for the rest of your life. This means choosing brown rice instead of white rice, whole-wheat or brown-rice pasta, quinoa, whole-wheat crackers and cereals, and so on. For more information on whole grains see Chapter 8, Concept #22.

Grains are the food group where many of our patients run into trouble.

If you feel that whole-grain bread or whole-wheat pasta is a trigger food for you, and that you can't just eat one slice or one serving, remove it from your meal plan altogether. Such items as crackers, cereals, or snack-based foods are very easy to overeat, and before starting on this plan you often paired them with other carbohydrates: for example, cereal and milk. Both are carbohydrates, and this pairing will not keep you full.

It may in fact make you hungrier! **If you've had trouble overeating snack foods or cereals in the past, avoid these types of grains completely.** Your body and brain need carbohydrates, but you can get sufficient carbohydrates from fruit or berries. **Grains are not a required part of your meal plan and do not supply nutrients that you can't get from protein, vegetables, and berries.** While grains have been a problem for many in our program, those participants who limited or avoided grains during and after their program reported greater success in both weight loss and weight maintenance.

For your meal plan, we measure grains and starchy vegetables in approximately 60-100 calorie servings and include only ONE per day. This is an easy rule to remember. Memorize this sentence to help yourself out:

Grains are tasty but can lead you astray. Limit them to one per day.

One hundred calories is usually equivalent to one slice of whole-grain bread. So, at a meal, you can have half a sandwich, but not a whole sandwich, because a whole sandwich would be two servings of grains. If you eat two servings of grains at a meal, it could cause your hunger and cravings to return. For cooked whole grains like brown rice, wild rice, quinoa etc., 100 calories is equal to a half cup cooked. You must check calorie counts and serving sizes for starchy vegetables, because they vary and are not standard at 100 calories. Refer to the serving size list in the beginning of this stage, and make sure to measure these items when including them.

When reintroducing grains, the trick to prevent cravings and weight gain is to introduce only 100 calories of grains every other day for the first week. As your comfort level improves, and if you're not experiencing hunger cravings, bloating, or distress, feel free to include one grain serving per day. While you're focusing on weight loss, never exceed one whole-grain serving, or 100 calories of whole grains or starchy vegetables per day. Over consuming grains is a surefire way to bring those hunger cravings back with a vengeance.

If you want to include your grain serving at breakfast, remember the limit on grains of 100 calories per day. You can choose a half cup cooked oatmeal, which is your one whole-grain serving for the entire day, but make sure you add protein and a heart-healthy fat. An example would be to add one cup nonfat Greek yogurt and 12 almonds to the half cup cooked oatmeal for a well-balanced breakfast that also includes grains.

Do not introduce grains in at snack times.

Many snacks are not high enough in protein to balance out a serving of grains, and 100-calorie portions of snack foods are often very small. Cheese and crackers sounds like a balanced snack, but beware! Crackers can trigger your reward center, and you may end up eating too many, which can cause hunger and cravings.

For lunch and dinner meals, your carbohydrate choices have expanded, but you still may only choose one carbohydrate serving per meal and one grain per day (which counts as your carbohydrate).

Know that grains are not a required food group. If introducing grains makes you hungry, tired, or gives you digestive problems, take them out of your meal plan. The second important issue with introduction of grains occurs when dining out. The rule is simple: When dining out, avoid grains. Bread served at restaurants is rarely whole grain and tends to be calorie dense. Furthermore, most of you can't stop at one slice (or one roll or one piece of garlic bread). For such items as rice or potatoes, restaurants will often serve significantly more food than you need. Even if you plan to only eat a small portion of the item, you'll undoubtedly consume more than a half cup, and that giant pasta or potato serving will lead to spikes in your blood sugar, causing the return of those hunger cravings.

When dining out, we recommend avoiding grains.

For healthy ways to dine out on ethnic foods, for example, Asian, Indian, or Hispanic, be sure to see Appendix L.

Grains aren't a required part of your nutrition, even though your previous dietary habits have taught you otherwise. The goal with this meal plan is to help you lose weight in a healthy manner, and if grains make you feel bad or make you hungry, remove them immediately.

In Stage 7 we introduce a new concept called the plate model. The plate model is a basic tool to teach you how to plan meals and show you what your plate should look like. The plate model will be a vital tool when you move towards weight maintenance. With the plate model, a third of your plate should be protein, a third should be your nonstarchy vegetable servings, and the final third should be your ONE carbohydrate choice. Following this model ensures that you maintain your protein and vegetable intake and control your carbohydrates as well.

Plates have also grown over the years. Be sure your plate is a 9 inch-diameter one, not the 14 inch, platter-sized one in common use.
This may come as a bit of a shock to you.

Here's a snapshot of what the plate looks like. We'll go into more detail regarding the plate model, once we reach maintenance.

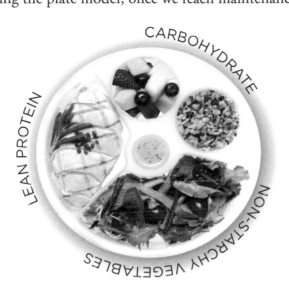

Good luck with Stage 7, and remember, *ONLY one grain per day.* *You can have one grain serving at either breakfast, lunch, or dinner, and it counts as your carbohydrate serving.*

Stage 7 includes whole-grain breads, cooked whole grains, whole-grain cereals and crackers, and starchy vegetables.

Servings: 1 serving per day for men and women

Calorie range: 60-100 calories per serving

For crackers, snack foods, or cereals, refer to the label on the package to determine the portion size that yields 100 calories.

All of these items are carbohydrates.

Serving sizes:

- Whole-grain bread: 1 serving = 1 slice or 100 calories

- Cooked whole grains: 1 serving = ½ cup cooked or 100 calories

- Cereals and whole-grain snacks: 1 serving = 100 calories

249

- Starchy vegetables: 1 serving = 60-100 calories

    ~ Corn: 1 serving = ½ cup

    ~ Peas: 1 serving = ½ cup

    ~ Potatoes, yams, sweet potato: 1 serving = 14 ounce potato cooked, or ½ cup mashed

    ~ Winter squash: 1 serving = ½ cup cubed

        * Examples: Acorn, butternut, pumpkin

SHOPPING LIST

Stage 7 includes whole-grain bread, cooked whole grains, whole-grain crackers, snacks and cereals, starchy vegetables.

Whole-grain bread

Here are the guidelines to look for when selecting a whole-grain bread:

- 3 grams or more of fiber per serving

- 3 grams or less of sugar per serving

- Look for the word "whole" in the first ingredient

- Avoid items with "enriched" in the first ingredient

- Approximately 100 calories per serving, containing 15-20 grams carbohydrate

Here are some whole-grain bread brands that fit within those guidelines. Remember to read the nutrition labels and look for the word "whole" in the first ingredient.

Examples:

☐ Oroweat Light 100 percent Whole Wheat Bread

☐ Oroweat Sandwich Thins

☐ Ezekiel Bread

☐ Franz 100 percent Whole Wheat Bread

☐ Dave's Killer Bread (Thin Sliced)

☐ La Tortilla Factory Whole Wheat Tortillas

☐ Flatout Bread

☐ Mission Low Carb Whole Wheat Tortillas

☐ Franz Mini whole wheat bagels

☐ Thomas Light English muffins

Cooked whole grains

Here are the guidelines to help you select a cooked grain that is a whole grain. Remember to be wary of wild rice varieties, as they may be a blend of whole grain and non-whole-grain items. If the food has a nutrition label, refer to it for more accurate nutrition facts.

Serving size for ½ cup cooked

Examples:

☐ Brown rice (long, short, or Basmati)　　☐ Millet

☐ Whole-wheat couscous　　☐ Amaranth

☐ Quinoa　　☐ Whole-wheat pasta

☐ Steel-cut oats　　☐ Brown-rice pasta

☐ Wild rice

☐ Barley

☐ Bulgur

Meal Ideas:

- ½ cup whole-wheat couscous with 4 ounces shrimp and 1½ cups asparagus

- ½ cup whole-wheat pasta with 4 ounces chicken sausage or turkey meatballs combined with ½ cup chopped bell pepper, ½ cup onions, and ½ cup tomatoes

- ½ cup quinoa with 1½ cups stir-fried mixed vegetables and chopped chicken

Whole-grain crackers and cereals

Crackers and cereals can be a trigger food for many people and also pose difficulties with portion control. These items are not a required part of your meal plan. They should only be included if they are truly whole grain, in small quantities, and always paired with protein or healthy fat. Here are the guidelines to help you make healthy choices.

☐ Whole-grain snack examples:

☐ Crackers: 100 calorie serving

☐ Ak-mak crackers

☐ TLC crackers

☐ Health Valley Low Fat Whole Wheat Crackers

☐ Wasa Crackers

☐ Mary's Gone Crackers

☐ Other snacks: check labels, serving sizes vary

☐ Whole-wheat matzos

☐ Whole-wheat pretzels (Snyder's)

☐ 100-calorie bags of popcorn

☐ Newman's Own Light Popcorn

☐ Van's Multi-Grain Toaster Waffles

Whole-grain cereal examples:

- ☐ Cold cereal: 100-calorie serving (less than 9 grams sugar, at least 3 grams fiber)
- ☐ Kellogg's All Bran
- ☐ Barbara's Shredded Spoonfuls
- ☐ Barbara's Oatios
- ☐ Barbara's Puffins Multigrain
- ☐ Kashi Go Lean or Good Friends
- ☐ Nature's Path Flax Plus
- ☐ General Mills Multi Grain Cheerios
- ☐ Post Grape Nuts
- ☐ Shredded Wheat
- ☐ Hot cereal: ½ cup cooked serving
- ☐ Arrowhead Mills
- ☐ Bob's Red Mill
- ☐ Hodgson Mill
- ☐ Nature's Path
- ☐ Quaker Oats (rolled or steel cut)

STAGE 7

Women 1,100-1,400 calories

BREAKFAST	CALORIES	FAT (g)
4 ounces very lean protein	140	0-4
2 heart-healthy fat servings *(see list for options)*	90	10
1 cup berries OR ½ cup fruit	60-80	0
Choose ONE of the choices listed below:		
1 serving of a whole-grain item	100	0
Breakfast Shake Alternatives		

LUNCH	CALORIES	FAT (g)
4 ounces very lean/lean protein OR 3 ounces very lean or lean protein plus 1 ounce cheese	140-220	0-12
1 heart-healthy fat servings *(add to very lean protein only)*	45	5
3 or more servings nonstarchy vegetables	45	0
Choose ONE of the carbohydrate choices listed below:		
1 cup berries, ½ cup fruit, ½ cup nonfat or low-fat flavored yogurt, 1 cup nonfat or low-fat milk, ½ cup cooked beans OR 1 serving whole-grain or starchy vegetable	60-100	0-3

SNACK *(1 per day between lunch and dinner)*	CALORIES	FAT (g)
2 light string cheeses plus ½ cup fruit	180	5
¼ cup hummus plus ½ cup mixed vegetables	130	4-6
2 ounces very lean protein plus 1 cup berries	130	0-2
20/20 LifeStyles High Protein Dry Powder Shake plus 1 cup berries *(NO peanut butter)*	260	0

DINNER	CALORIES	FAT (g)
4 ounces very lean/lean protein OR 3 ounces very lean or lean protein plus 1 ounce cheese	140-220	0-12
1 heart-healthy fat servings *(add to very lean protein only)*	45	5
3 or more servings nonstarchy vegetables	45	0
Choose ONE of the carbohydrate choices listed below:		
1 cup berries, ½ cup fruit, ½ cup nonfat or low-fat flavored yogurt, 1 cup nonfat or low-fat milk, ½ cup cooked beans OR 1 serving of whole grain or starchy vegetable *(only if you have not had your grain serving today)*	60-100	0-3

SAMPLE MENU

DAY 1

BREAKFAST:

- 20/20 LifeStyles High Protein Dry Powder Shake

- 1 tablespoon almond butter

- 1 cup blueberries

LUNCH:

- 4 ounces chicken breast baked with 1 teaspoon oil for cooking

- ½ cup cooked low-sodium black beans

- 3 tablespoons fresh salsa

- Make a slaw with:

  - 1 cup sliced jicama

  - ½ cup sliced carrots

SNACK:

- 20/20 LifeStyles Protein Bar

DINNER:

- 4 ounces baked pork tenderloin

- 1½ cups broccoli

- ½ cup cooked quinoa

DAY 2

BREAKFAST:

- ½ cup oatmeal cooked in water, topped with 5 chopped walnut halves
- 2 whole eggs scrambled with 2 egg whites

LUNCH:

- 4 ounces baked salmon
- 1½ cups steamed green beans
- 1 cup strawberries

SNACK:

- 1 cup flavored nonfat Greek yogurt
- 1-2 tablespoons nuts or seeds

DINNER:

- 4 ounces grilled chicken breast
- Make a salad with:
    - 1½ cups romaine lettuce
    - ½ cup tomato
    - ½ cup sliced cucumber
    - 2 tablespoons low-fat dressing
- 1 cup raspberries

DAY 3

BREAKFAST:

- 6 egg whites scrambled with 1 whole egg

- 1 tennis-ball-sized apple

- 2 teaspoons peanut butter

LUNCH:

- Make a sandwich with:

    ~ 4 ounces canned tuna mixed

    ~ 1 tablespoon reduced-fat mayo

    ~ 1 slice (100 calories) whole-grain bread

    ~ 2 romaine lettuce leaves

    ~ 2-3 tomato slices

- 1 cup carrots

SNACK:

- 2 low-fat cheese sticks

- ½ cup grapes

DINNER:

- 4 ounces grilled chicken breast

- Make a salad with:

    ~ 1½ cups spinach

    ~ ½ cup garbanzo beans

- ~ ½ cup chopped radish

- ~ ¼ cup chopped carrots

- ~ ¼ cup chopped tomato

- ~ 2 tablespoons low-fat salad dressing

STAGE 7

Men 1,300-1,700 calories

BREAKFAST	CALORIES	FAT (g)
4 ounces very lean protein	140	0-4
2 heart-healthy fat servings *(see list for options)*	90	10
1 cup berries OR ½ cup fruit	60-80	0
OR		
1 serving of a whole-grain item	100	0
OR		
Breakfast Shake Alternatives		

LUNCH	CALORIES	FAT (g)
6 ounces very lean/lean protein OR 5 ounces very lean or lean protein plus 1 ounce cheese	210-330	0-18
1 heart-healthy fat servings *(add to very lean protein only)*	45	5
3 or more servings nonstarchy vegetables	45	0
Choose ONE of the carbohydrate choices listed below:		
1 cup berries, ½ cup fruit, ½ cup nonfat or low-fat flavored yogurt, 1 cup nonfat or low-fat milk, ½ cup cooked beans OR 1 serving whole-grain or starchy vegetable	60-100	0-3

SNACK *(2 per day between lunch and dinner): Choose ONE of these options for your snack.*	CALORIES	FAT (g)
2 light string cheeses plus ½ cup fruit	180	5
¼ cup hummus plus ½ cup mixed vegetables	130	4-6
2 ounces very lean protein plus 1 cup berries	130	0-2
20/20 LifeStyles High Protein Dry Powder Shake plus 1 cup berries *(NO peanut butter)*	260	0

DINNER	CALORIES	FAT (g)
6 ounces very lean/lean protein OR 5 ounces very lean or lean protein plus 1 ounce cheese	210-330	0-18
1 heart-healthy fat servings *(add to very lean protein only)*	45	5
3 or more servings nonstarchy vegetables	45	0
Choose ONE of the carbohydrate choices listed below:		
1 cup berries, ½ cup fruit, ½ cup nonfat or low-fat flavored yogurt, 1 cup nonfat or low-fat milk, ½ cup cooked beans OR 1 serving of whole grain or starchy vegetable *(only if you have not had your grain serving today)*	60-100	0-3

Breakfast ideas:

- Layer 1 cup of nonfat plain Greek yogurt with a 100 calorie portion of whole-grain cereal and 1 tablespoon chopped nuts or seeds to make a parfait
- One whole-grain waffle (100 calories) with a side of 2 ounces low-sodium turkey sausage and 4 scrambled egg whites topped with 1 tablespoon natural peanut butter

Starchy vegetables

For starchy vegetables such as corn, peas, potatoes, sweet potatoes, and winter squash, even though we call them vegetables, we treat them like a carbohydrate. Be very mindful of measuring with these items to be sure you don't exceed the 100-calorie recommendation. If you find that these items trigger you to eat more or cause hunger, it's best to avoid them altogether.

> *One serving of starchy vegetables is 60-100 calories, approximately 15-20 grams carbohydrate, and counts as a carbohydrate food choice.*

The foods in this category are VERY dangerous. It's best not to regularly include them in your meal plan, but if you do, follow these guidelines for portion size. If the food has a nutrition label, refer to it for more accurate nutrition facts.

Serving suggestions:

In restaurants or in traditional home cooking, starchy vegetables are often fried or prepared with butter, sugar, maple syrup, sour cream, cheese, and other high-calorie toppings. However, there are healthy and tasty alternative ways to prepare these vegetables.

- Use low-sodium chicken broth instead of butter on mashed potatoes.

- Top ½ cup puréed winter squash with cinnamon, nutmeg, and a splash of orange juice. Top with walnut or pecan halves and bake for a healthy carbohydrate plus fat side dish.

- Bake a small potato or sweet potato spears on baking sheet coated with PAM spray at 400° F. for 30-35 minutes (a serving is 4 ounces). Sprinkle with herbs or spices such as paprika, pumpkin pie spice, chili seasoning, or garlic powder before baking for even more flavor.

- Top a small baked potato with fat-free plain or Greek yogurt, salsa, or low-fat cheese instead of sour cream or butter.

- Sprinkle corn or peas on a mixed green salad.

SAMPLE MENU

DAY 1

BREAKFAST:

- 20/20 LifeStyles High Protein Dry Powder Shake

- 1 tablespoon almond butter

- 1 cup blueberries

SNACK:

- 20/20 LifeStyles Protein Bar

LUNCH:

- 6 ounces chicken breast baked with 1 teaspoon oil for cooking

- ½ cup cooked low-sodium black beans

- 3 tablespoons salsa

- Make a slaw with:

   - ½ cup sliced jicama

   - ½ cup sliced carrots

SNACK:

- 6 ounces flavored nonfat Greek yogurt

- 1-2 tablespoons nuts or seeds

DINNER:

- 6 ounces baked pork tenderloin

- 1 cup steamed broccoli

- ½ cup cooked quinoa

DAY 2

BREAKFAST:

- ½ cup oatmeal cooked in water, topped with 5 chopped walnut halves
- 2 whole eggs scrambled with 2 egg whites

SNACK:

- 2 tablespoons hummus
- 1 cup carrots

LUNCH:

- 6 ounces salmon
- 1½ cups steamed green beans
- ½ cup cut-up mixed fruit

SNACK:

- 2 hardboiled eggs
- 1 tennis-ball-sized apple

DINNER:

- 6 ounces grilled chicken breast
- Make a salad with:
    - ½ cup garbanzo beans
    - 1½ cups romaine lettuce
    - ½ cup chopped tomato
    - ½ cup sliced cucumber
    - 2 tablespoons low-fat dressing

264

DAY 3

BREAKFAST:

- 6 egg whites scrambled with 1 whole egg

- 1 tennis-ball-sized apple

- 2 teaspoons peanut butter

SNACK:

- 20/20 LifeStyles Protein Bar

LUNCH:

- Make a sandwich with:

  ~ 6 ounces canned tuna mixed

  ~ 1 tablespoon reduced fat mayo

  ~ 100 calorie portion of whole-grain bread

  ~ 2 romaine lettuce leaves

  ~ 2-3 tomato slices

- 1 cup carrots

SNACK:

- 2 low-fat cheese sticks

- ½ cup grapes

DINNER:

- 6 ounces grilled chicken breast

- Make a salad with:

  ~ 1½ cups spinach

- ~ ½ cup chopped radish

- ~ ¼ cup chopped carrots

- ~ ¼ cup chopped tomato

- ~ 2 tablespoons low-fat salad dressing

- 1 cup raspberries

EXERCISE PLAN: I AM AMAZING

You're now in great shape. For many of you this will be the best physical condition of your entire adult life until now. Now's the time to reach out and try something you've dreamed about, something from your own personal bucket list. Ever wanted to run a marathon, climb a mountain, go on a bicycle tour, or join an adult sports league? Now you can do it. GO FOR IT!

Exercise Will Be As Follows

Level 1: Low fitness- Running or hill-walking for 15 minutes, then fast walking for 10 minutes. Repeat twice for a total of 50 minutes, at least 5 days per week. Keep your pace at a level to reach your optimum heart rate range (65-85 percent of your maximum).

Level 2: Moderate fitness- Running or hill-walking for 40 minutes, then high-speed walking for 10 minutes, at least 5 days per week. Keep your heart rate at optimum level (65-85 percent of your maximum).

Level 3: High fitness- Running 6 miles, 4 days per week, and 8 miles, 1 day per week. For an extra, 6th day workout, run 6 miles. Continue running gradual hills. Heart rate at optimum level (65-85 percent of your maximum). Continue timing your runs. You should now be close to 6 miles in 45 minutes.

All levels: Keep wearing your pedometer when not exercising, and keep your steps at 6,000 per day, excluding your exercise routine.

LIFESTYLE PLAN:
REASONABLE EXPECTATIONS

You want this to be the last time you ever have to lose a substantial amount of weight. But that doesn't mean that you won't have difficulties in the future. The physical, environmental, and educational issues that caused you to gain weight in the first place are still there. You're bombarded with advertising for unhealthy lifestyles, and every time you go into a restaurant or food store, you see and smell those foods.

Now is the time to start thinking about your long-term plan, how you will manage your weight and your health for the rest of your life. Back in Chapter 1 we discussed self-acceptance and that you're a fallible human being, just like the rest of us. Having accepted that, you must now accept the idea that you will do nothing we have laid out in this book perfectly. You'll occasionally lose control of your time and skip exercise or eat foods off your plan. You'll occasionally lapse into unhealthy eating. And, as a result, you'll occasionally gain some of your weight back[31].

You need to understand "lapse and relapse." A lapse is an unplanned mistake or slip you make in following your plan. It's a single event, in which you lose self-control and then re-establish it. A relapse is a significant loss of your self-control (a whole series of lapses or slips) that lead to you giving up and starting to regain your lost weight or the metabolic disorder that you had put into remission.

---

31. *See videos on Lapse and Relapse and How to Stay Motivated for Life in the Lifestyles Series in Appendix J.*

You need to learn to manage lapses, so that they don't turn into relapse. Let's look at the cause of relapses-high risk situations.

- A major increase in your stress due to work, family, or finances

- Having negative emotions like depression, anger, and fear

- Travelling

- Spending time with friends and family, who love to eat unhealthy foods

- Eating out

- Holidays

- Parties and celebrations

- Major change in your life: marriage, divorce, having a child, moving, changing jobs

- A crisis with your parents or siblings

- Injury and illness

RELAPSE PREVENTION PROTOCOL

The first step in not letting these situations destroy your health is to rapidly identify them as high-risk situations. Next you need to launch into your relapse prevention protocol:

Forgive yourself: going back through self-acceptance, self-respect, and self-love. Remember, it's much easier to do good things for yourself when you love yourself.

Analyze what you did wrong: what you did, and why you did it. Don't settle for easy answers like "I just wanted to" or "I don't know." You may have to get out that paper, laptop, or tablet to find the real reasons.

Create a plan: You have this book, and you have a stepwise process for breaking the destructive eating patterns. Use that process. Remember, going back to Stage 2 of the meal plan is your first-aid kit. Use it!

Use visualization to rehearse your plan: Be sure you see yourself back on plan and feel very good about that.

Create a plan to use the next time: You will find yourself in that same high-risk situation, so you don't relapse again.

If you follow these instructions, you will have taken a potentially disastrous situation and turned it into a learning experience that will help you in the future.

Now, you're moving forward with your lifestyle. At this point you should be adapting what you've learned in this book to your daily life. From this point on, we'll begin to focus on what happens after you've reached your goal weight and how you will make your lifestyle changes permanent.

CHAPTER 13

WELCOME TO YOUR FUTURE-MAINTAINING YOUR WEIGHT LOSS AND YOUR NEW HEALTH

MY BODY WAS A TIME BOMB
Arthur, age 26

Looking back on it all, with what I know now, I'm truly amazed that I survived what I put myself through.

Here I was, a young guy with a good job at a large software company but so completely focused on my work that I didn't understand what the rest of my life was about.

Imagine someone 25 years old who had high blood pressure, extremely high cholesterol, suffered from chronic depression, and weighed 236 pounds. That was me.

To complete that picture, add the fact that I was a heavy smoker. I also consumed literally gallons of diet soda each day, and with all that nicotine and caffeine intake, I was sleeping erratically-between 2 to 4 hours on week nights.

I was young and thought I was bullet proof. This was the way we'd all lived when I was at college. Bodies were something to be used and abused, and burning the candle at both ends was a way of life.

The stress at work became a huge factor, but it was my lifestyle that had created the sleeplessness.

I considered myself a work-warrior, and I would tough it out while on the job, giving it my all, but then I would hit my favorite restaurant

271

on my way home and pig out as a reward for having made it through another long, hard day. No matter how much overtime I worked, I would schedule my departure from the office so that I could get to that restaurant before it closed.

To make things worse, I would never go to sleep until my "smoking day" was done, meaning until I had my fill of nicotine for that 24-hour period, which sometimes meant going to bed as early as 10:00 p.m. and other times as late as 4:00 a.m., depending on when my body seemed satiated on cigarettes. This erratic schedule in my sleep hours was constant, but I made it to work on time every morning at 8 a.m.

That was my Monday-through-Friday routine.

On weekends, I was so exhausted that I would spend both days in bed, sleeping 10 or more hours each day to try to make up for the rest of the week. To make things worse, I would frequently buy the largest pizza I could find and have it in bed with me so that I could snack on it whenever I awoke to eat and watch TV.

What truly amazes me about that phase in my life and my deteriorating health is that I didn't consider my lifestyle all that bad. I suppose that was because you never really see how damaging things are, until someone who's qualified takes the time to point it out to you.

When I came to the 20/20 LifeStyles program, I learned how I could change my behavior and my lifestyle. I had tried to change my habits before, but I had always failed.

I grew up in Brazil, and several years ago, when a friend and co-worker sponsored me for employment, I came to the United States permanently. Before that, while I'd attended college in the United States, I'd been back-and-forth between the two countries several times. And as a result of my travels, a noticeable pattern took shape. When I was home in Brazil, since my parents were both slim and my mother's cooking was very healthy, I tended to keep my weight down. But when I stayed in the United States for any length of time, I'd balloon to a larger size-something I attributed to the American diet-but my love of fast food played a big part. During my college years in Brazil, I worked out more, and even though my weight went up and down for some time, on average, I was able to maintain what I considered my "normal" weight, around 167 pounds.

Once I became employed in the United States I tried to quit smoking on a number of occasions, and I even went through several smoking cessation programs, but that never worked for me. I hired a personal trainer to try and stay in shape. That also had no lasting effect. So, it wasn't that I was unaware of my unhealthy lifestyle, I just found myself unable to change. Yet after repeated failures, and after becoming fully immersed in my work, the stress was running my life. Any progress I had made for better health disappeared, and my food, exercise, and sleep habits just got worse.

The doctors at 20/20 LifeStyles, along with my fitness trainer, dietitian, and lifestyle counselors, fully understood my problem. They viewed my issues not just as weight-loss challenges, but also as lifestyle challenges. They seemed to live my struggle with me-supportive at an emotional level, feeling my pain and celebrating my victories. Their constant care and support had a huge effect, and I began to feel like a different person.

Obviously, the chemical imbalances I'd created with my addiction to cigarettes, soda, food, and lack of sleep were much to blame for my unhealthy life, and correcting those habits and behaviors certainly meant a lot, but it was the mental change caused by 20/20 LifeStyles that made the difference.

I began to feel so good about myself that I intuitively didn't want to hurt my body anymore. If you want to call that self-love, I think you can. Initially, I hadn't looked at it that way, but I've since learned that

I'm worth it. Keeping the weight off and treating my body with respect is something I continue to do, because it helps me be happy and healthy.

And in regard to smoking, knowing the damage it would do to my new body, I can't imagine ever doing that again. Going forward in my new life, I keep the lessons I learned in the 20/20 LifeStyles program at the top of my mind. I never forget what a physical and emotional wreck I was at 25 years old. And I'll do whatever is necessary to keep my self-respect, self-love, and respect for my body.

Arthur was so pleased with his new life and new body that he wanted to do whatever was necessary to sustain his newfound health and happiness. He recognized that keeping the lessons at the top of his mind was essential.

CONCEPT #23
How To keep Your Focus

If you've followed the directions and advice outlined in this book, you've become a new person. You look and feel wonderful. Your friends, family, and workgroup are amazed at your success. You're buying clothes that you believed would never look good on you, and you're engaging in physical activities at a level that amazes you. Being this "new you" is an invigorating and powerful experience, and because of your positive changes you're energized and focused on what you've learned. As rejuvenated as you feel, though, keep in mind that the newness and excitement of your feelings won't last forever.

As challenging as losing your weight and getting into great physical shape might have been for you, that was actually the easier part of your journey to lifelong health. That's right, losing weight and getting fit was the easy part. The hard part is keeping it that way.

At some point in the future, this book will be collecting dust on a back shelf, and you'll take the newness of your weight, looks, and fitness for granted. The factor in your life that will not have changed is the unhealthy food environment we all live in. The fast-food restaurants will still be there, the unhealthy foods will still be there, and the overweight Americans happily eating all those foods will still be there.

The challenge is, then, how to stay motivated for life. How do you keep the positive motivation that has given you this great success you now enjoy?

To understand that, let's look at an example of how motivation works. Imagine you're teaching a little girl something completely new and different, such as how to swim. As the teacher, you'd encourage the child to make her feel at ease, compliment her on her progress, and make suggestions to help her improve. You'd show delight in her progress and be very accepting of her failures. Does this encouragement sound like anything you may have read earlier in this book?

The combination of self-acceptance, self-respect, and self-love IS motivation.

Remember, having a negative attitude-that is, emphasizing what you've done wrong-is de-motivating. So, now that you've changed yourself into this new and healthy person, remember to continue changing the things you need to improve, without condemning yourself for having done them wrong in the first place. That means you need to accept the responsibility without accepting the blame. Self-acceptance means acknowledging your faults, by saying "Yes, I did that," but rejecting the idea that you're a failure, a bad or a weak person, or that you're out of control.

By now you've learned that it's difficult to stay motivated, and there are a thousand excuses for you to lose your motivation. So here are some techniques to keep you motivated:

1. Create yellow and red light points for your weight

Often, your weight gain will actually occur a few days after you've lost control of your eating. That means you may have lapsed into disordered eating a few days before you start to see the scale move. So, the best real-time indicator that you're having problems is, of course, your meal tracker.

To prevent more serious problems, you must create firm weight points to indicate that your motivation has been seriously eroded. We call these warning points the "yellow light" and "red light" weights. Your yellow-light weight point should be 3 pounds above your maintenance weight, and your red-light point should be 5 pounds above your maintenance weight.

If you reach your yellow-light point, you MUST take corrective action as discussed earlier in this chapter. If you reach your red-light point, you need to rally your support group and all of your self-help techniques to get you back on track, because you're in real trouble.

More detail on the emergency actions you need to take are in Technique 2.

2. Write a contract with yourself

There is something affirming about writing it down on paper that makes you realize you deserve to be happy, healthy, and need to love yourself. You've worked very hard to get to this point, and you deserve to keep the weight off and enjoy increased energy, flexibility, and strength. When you write your contract, be specific. Don't just write, "I promise to eat healthy and go to the gym at least four to five times a week." Instead write, "I will meal-track on my 20/20 app 3 days per week, and if I lapse, I will track every meal for the next month. Also, I will admit the lapse to my support people to give me accountability. I will exercise 4-5 times per week, no matter what really good excuses I have for not doing it. I'll continue to exercise with my workout buddies. If I start missing exercise sessions, I will also admit that to my support people. I will wear my pedometer at least 3 days a week, so I can keep my steps to at least 6,000 a day. I will weigh myself daily, and if I hit my red-light number, I will take emergency action. I will track every meal for a month, I will open this book and begin reading it over again, I will go back to Stage 2 on my food plan and stay there for at least one week to eliminate my food cravings, and I will clean the junk food out of the house ."

You get the idea. Now, do it. Sit down and write that contract!

3. Use visualization

Visualization is a wonderful technique to sustain motivation. We discussed visualization in Chapter 6. It's been said that the famous basketball player, Michael Jordan, visualized his shots many times before he attempted them. He said that when he actually went to make them, he felt as if he'd made them many times before. You can achieve that same success by changing your habits through visualization. When you visualize yourself successfully performing a new habit, such as turning down the hors d'oeuvres tray or ordering sparkling water instead of alcohol, you will automatically perform that new habit when faced with the actual situation.

To help get you started, here's a visualization exercise that will enable you to stay motivated. Remember, to execute this properly, you need to choose a quiet and comfortable location where you wont' be interrupted.

Now, sit back, relax, and see yourself at a transition place in your life. Your wedding, retirement, 50th anniversary, child's graduation, etc. Visualize yourself being at normal weight, fit, and healthy. See yourself at the dinner, banquet, or party that goes along with this event. Now see yourself passing up the bread, pastries, wine, pasta, and other high-calorie foods and enjoying a healthy meal. Let yourself feel the positive feelings, comfort, and security this gives you. Look back on the years that you've maintained your health and fitness and see that it was truly worth all the effort. Be specific in visualizing your details.

It's also a good idea to visualize the dangers and plot a course through them. Visualize the tempting food and drink, other people enjoying their unhealthy eating and drinking, etc. Now, visualize yourself enjoying the event, friends, family, and the healthy food and drink options available-and, finally, feeling great at the end of the event.

4. Weigh yourself daily, or at least weekly

Avoiding the scale is a sure sign of imminent relapse. If you find you haven't weighed in for over a week, immediately assess the need to go to your yellow or red light plan.

5. Beware of "portion bloat"

Funny how when you stop weighing and measuring, your food portions start to expand. Your carbohydrate portion, which was meant to be ½ cup or the size of a tennis ball, starts to grow and grow until soon it's bigger than your plate. To avoid this shift in your perceptions, at least one week out of the month go back to weighing and measuring your food. It will help you keep focused.

6. Avoid slipping back to those old eating habits

Slipping back to your old eating habits is deadly. Remember, lifestyle change is the secret to success, and falling back into your old lifestyle is the fast track to disaster. Fast foods, foods rich in sugar, fat, and salt, lots of carbohydrates, eating whenever and wherever you feel like it are signs of total relapse.

7. Stay in control of your time

If you allow your time management to get sloppy, pretty soon there'll be no time to eat healthy, exercise, or sleep. Beyond that, poor time management will increase your stress level and cortisol level. Now your cravings return, and since you've made no time to eat well, and you didn't prepare in advance, you'll wind up eating what's convenient. But, fortunately, your experience using the 20/20 LifeStyles plan has taught you how to keep your time in control. Go back to Chapter 11 and read the time-management section again.

8. Never skip workouts

There are so many CONVINCING reasons for skipping workouts! Throughout this book we've recommended that you get a workout buddy. We know that this can be difficult at times. It may be hard to find someone who has the same schedule as you. Your workout buddy may be ill or injured. Your workout buddy might move or get a new job. But if you temporarily lose your workout buddy, you can still take steps to help keep you on track. Sign up for a class at your local health club, school, or community center. By signing up for a class, you'll have a schedule to keep you on track. If you know you're going to be in a spinning, step, or total body makeover class from 6 to 7 p.m., and the teacher is expecting you to be there, you will be there. Join a sports team-something like soccer that involves substantial activity. Knowing that your teammates are expecting you will help keep you on track. Learn a new active hobby such as rock climbing, racquetball, squash, or cross-country skiing. Showing up for your instructor or class will be good motivation for you. You can also get a personal trainer to help keep you accountable.

9. Use the 20/20 LifeStyles online app

We mentioned the 20/20 LifeStyles app in Chapter 9. www.2020lifestyles.com/get-started/get-started-online/track-it.aspx.

This is an excellent resource for your continued success.

Remember, there are more than 60 educational videos, recipes, and other aids to help you with your 20/20 LifeStyles plan and your continued successful maintenance.

After reading this book, the 20/20 application will make perfect sense to you, and meal tracking should become second nature. In your tracker, or on the 20/20 LifeStyles website, under the Resources and Tools tab you'll find two very important tools to help you maintain your weight. The first is the Weekly Dietitian Review. Since meal tracking is now a habit, the Weekly Dietitian Review adds an extra dose of accountability and guidance to a task that you're already doing daily. One of our registered dietitians will review your meal tracker each week, providing comments, feedback, and goals to help you continue to either lose or maintain your weight. Think of this as having your own personal dietitian reviewing your progress each week. This is also a great platform for you to communicate your questions or needs to your dietitian. The second tool is called Ask An Expert. This is perfect for those instances where you're dining out and don't know what to order, or have a nutrition question that you can't answer. This tool allows you to text a live dietitian or personal trainer with your question. You'll get answers to your questions in just minutes. Take advantage of these tools. Both are available through the Essentials Plus and Premium Packages. Get started now! www.2020lifestyles.com/get-started/get-started-online/pricing.aspx

It can take 2 years to firmly establish all the lifestyle or habit changes you have acquired during the plan. Remember, we talked about the gravity of your old lifestyle and how it continually tries to pull you back. We also talked about how you revert to the old habits when you are stressed or sleep deprived. After 2 years, you'll be established in your new lifestyle and habits. At that point, returning to the old ways will feel uncomfortably wrong, and the lifestyle you adopted as a result of this book will now be your old comfortable habit.

NUTRITION FOR LIFE

Congratulations! You've now reached the maintenance phase of your meal plan. This means that you've completed all 7 of the stages, have added back all the food groups, and reached your goal weight. Maintenance is all about continuing what you've learned through this process in regard to exercise, nutrition, and lifestyle for success in maintaining your new weight for the rest of your life.

What does maintenance really look like? Well, to begin with, maintenance is much more difficult than weight loss. During weight loss, you often refuse treats or alcohol easily, because you're on a food plan. What happens when you no longer have weight to lose?

Now, in case you're thinking, "Finally, I'm done with this plan," think again. The principles we've taught you regarding nutrition and nutrient balance still apply. What will change in maintenance is your total calorie intake. Once you reach your goal weight, you'll need to slowly increase your calories to stop losing and begin maintaining your weight. Let's review the plate model that we discussed in the previous chapter and learn how to transition into weight maintenance.

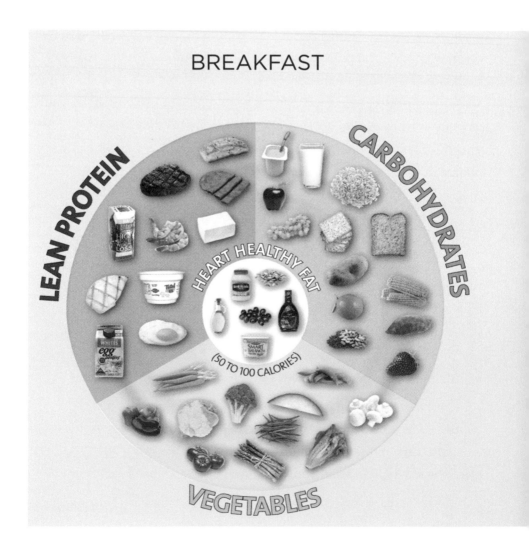

For breakfast, your plate will look very similar to the previous weeks. Know that many of our most successful clients continued to have a 20/20 LifeStyles Protein Shake with berries and peanut butter to start their morning routine for years after they've reached their goal weight. So, if the shakes are working for you, include them as a fast, balanced breakfast for the rest of your life!

For both men and women, whole food based breakfasts should include 4 or more ounces of protein, 2 healthy fat servings, as many vegetable servings as you would like, and only 1 carbohydrate.

PROTEIN:

Women: 4+ ounces of protein

Men: 4+ ounces of protein

Increase protein is a great way to increase your total calories for the meal, while still keeping you satiated. To increase calories, you may consume higher that the recommendations given above.

CARBOHYDRATES:

1 serving = 60-100 calories

Choose ONE:

- 1 cup berries
- ½ cup non-Greek yogurt
- ½ cup fruit
- 1 cup skim or 1 percent milk
- ½ cup beans

- ½ cup cooked whole grain
- 100 calories of whole grain cerial
- 1 slice of bread
- ½ cup of starchy vegetables

NON-STARCHY VEGETABLES: Unlimited

2 HEART HEALTHY FAT SERVINGS

Protein in the morning is crucial! So always make sure to have a protein-rich breakfast. What may change is choosing to have a grain-based food with your meal, such as a slice of whole-wheat toast instead of some other carbohydrate. If you use a grain serving at breakfast, make that your *only* carbohydrate for the meal. We have included vegetables on the breakfast plate, because they're a wonderful way to add volume and fiber without adding calories. Add some spinach to a morning protein shake, or bell peppers and onions to an omelet or scramble. To increase calories

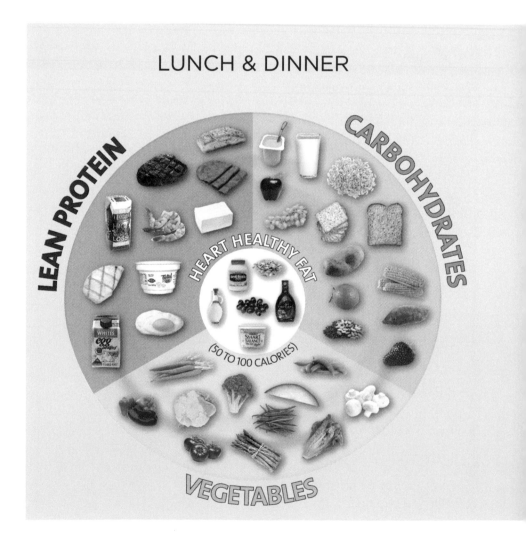

in your breakfast meal, increase your protein by 1-2 ounces and be sure to include 2 heart-healthy fat servings.

Let's take a look at your plate for lunch and dinner. You'll see that ⅓ of your plate is protein, ⅓ carbohydrates, ⅓ vegetables, which is identical to the weight-loss portion of your meal plan. For lunch and dinner, women aim for a minimum of 4-6 ounces of protein, and men aim for 6-8 ounces minimum. Include 2 heart-healthy fat servings at both lunch and dinner to provide an increase in calories. You may

PROTEIN:

Women: 4-6+ ounces of protein

Men: 6-8+ ounces of protein

Increase protein is a great way to increase your total calories for the meal, while still keeping you satiated. To increase calories, you may consume higher that the recommendations given above.

CARBOHYDRATES:

1 serving = 60-100 calories

Choose ONE:

- 1 cup berries
- ½ cup non-Greek yogurt
- ½ cup fruit
- 1 cup skim or 1 percent milk
- ½ cup beans
- ½ cup cooked whole grain
- 100 calories of whole grain cerial
- 1 slice of bread
- ½ cup of starchy vegetables

NON-STARCHY VEGETABLES: Unlimited

2 HEART HEALTHY FAT SERVINGS

Increase healthy fat servings is another way to increase calories, while keeping you satiated.

also increase calories with extra protein. **Do not add calories to your meal plan by adding more carbohydrates.** Choose one of the items listed above as your carbohydrate for the meal. We don't recommend increasing calories through carbohydrates, because, as we've said before, eating too much carbohydrate leads to hunger, cravings, and weight gain. So, for lunch and dinner, increase your calories through lean protein and healthy fats.

Fatty meats such as bacon, lamb, pork, beef ribs, or higher-fat steak cuts like prime rib or a ribeye will yield more calories than very lean and lean meats. Make sure to track these items, and omit the additional fat servings with the meal.

The last way to increase calories is through snacks. Snacks should always be balanced. Carbohydrates always need to be paired with a healthy fat or a protein. Adding an extra snack at mid-morning, for example, a small apple and 2 tablespoons of peanut butter, is an easy way to add about 250 calories to your meal plan. Another great way to add a balanced 100-200 calories to your day is 1 cup of carrots and 4 tablespoons of hummus. Just remember to avoid using grains as a snack. It's easy to eat too much of such items as crackers or cereals, and many times with those foods your snack won't have enough protein to balance out the carbohydrates. Also, unless you'll be awake for more than 4 hours after dinner, **do not add a second snack after dinner. If you go to bed within 4 hours of dinner, dinner should be your last food for the day.**

The plates shown above are very similar to the nutrition plan in Stage 7. That's because, in maintenance as well as in weight loss, calories need to be controlled, and we have to keep our bodies in chemical balance. Protein and vegetables will still be the key to keeping you full and satisfied. The only changes are your recommended calorie range and the flexibility within your plan.

To calculate your maintenance calorie range, you will need to calculate your basal metabolic rate (BMR)-the number of calories your body burns at rest. From there, you'll take into account exercise, and determine a target calorie range. Calorie recommendations will vary from person to person, based on your age, gender, height, weight, and activity level. Many of us overestimate how many calories we burn in a day, so it's very important to calculate your maintenance calorie range accurately.

The chart shown on the website listed below provides a good estimate of what your BMR may be. Look to the "kcal" column corresponding to your weight in kilograms to find your estimated BMR. To get your weight in kilograms, divide your weight in pounds by 2.2. www.ideal-weight-charts.com/calories-to-maintain-weight.html

This chart does not take into account age or height, so for more specific calculations, see the link or equation below. Here is a link to calculate your specific BMR, or you can find a simple BMR calculator online. www.bmrcalculator.org/

If you prefer to do it by hand, here is the equation:

MEN-BMR =10 x weight(kg)+6.25 x height(cm)-5 x age(y)+5

WOMEN-BMR =10 x weight(kg)+6.25 x height(cm)-5 x age(y)-161

Once you have your BMR, we need to take into account activity. So, multiply your BMR by 1.2 for low to moderate activity and by 1.4 for high activity levels.

This will give you a target for maintenance, which takes into account your activity level as well. For example, if you calculate your BMR to be 1,350 calories, your maintenance calorie range would be 1,620-1,890 per day, depending on your activity range. It's important that you calculate your approximate weight-maintenance range, because most people overestimate their maintenance range.

Let's take an example. Say you're a 39-year-old woman with a full-time job and a 10-year-old child. Your activity level is moderate plus. Your height is 5 feet 7, and you weigh 130 pounds. You go to www.bmrcalculator.org/, plug in your age, height, and weight and get a BMR of 1,300 calories per day. Now because you're fairly active, you multiply that by 1.3 to get 1,690. This is your APPROXIMATE maintenance daily calorie intake. At the completion of the weight-loss portion of the plan, you were eating 1,300 calories per day, so for Week One on maintenance, you would increase to 1,400 per day, Week Two to 1,500, and so on until your weight levels out. DO NOT IMMEDIATELY JUMP TO 1,690 PER DAY. Remember, this is an approximate calorie burn. Always start your increase a few hundred calories below the calculated approximation.

As you approach maintenance, your weight loss will begin to slow down. So, for most of you, maintenance will not make a very big difference in your nutrition plan.

To start increasing your calories, you need two sources of data: your tracker and your weight. To begin, start by increasing your calories by 100 per day. So if you are currently consuming 1,400 calories daily, increase your intake to 1,500 calories daily. Eat about 1,500 calories each day for a full week. The easiest way to do this is to add another 100-calorie snack, or extra protein, or a healthy fat serving to a meal. For example, ¼ avocado or 12 almonds is a quick way to add 2 healthy fat servings and increase calories slightly.

Once you've increased your intake by 100 calories daily, weigh yourself. If after a week your weight decreases further, increase by another 100 calories daily for the following week and continue until your weight remains constant. Hence, the next week would be 1,600 calories each day for the week. Then you would weigh yourself again to see if your weight went down, stayed stable, or went up. This gradual increase will help your body adjust to your new meal plan. Continue in this manner until you reach the calorie range where your weight stabilizes. Increased or decreased exercise may change your calorie needs, so you'll need to continue meal tracking, and weighing yourself regularly to ensure that your weight stays constant.

To maintain your weight, continued meal tracking and healthy eating habits are the most important pieces of your new healthy lifestyle. We've seen numerous clients lose weight, go back to their poor dietary habits, but maintain their weight only because of a strenuous workout regimen. The statement "You can't exercise off a bad diet" is true. Those individuals whose weight maintenance relied on large amounts of exercise to balance out a poor diet gained their weight back. Injuries, illness, time conflicts, etc., will get in the way of exercise at some point. Meal planning, tracking, and making healthy food choices should be your first priority when it comes to weight maintenance. At any time if you feel you are regaining weight, or struggling with tracking, always reach out for support from a dietitian. Sometimes increasing your accountability can help you keep your weight off for good.

Two items-a type of food and a type of beverage-we haven't yet discussed in any detail: dessert and alcohol. Once again, these two categories are unnecessary for your body's functioning. So, if you try alcohol or a dessert and find yourself becoming hungry, you must remove that item from your plan. Always use alcohol and dessert sparingly, and use them as your carbohydrate for the meal. So, instead of brown rice at dinner, you may have a glass of wine. Limit the portion of alcohol or dessert to 300 calories, and limit either to 1-2 times weekly. This means avoiding such high-sugar beverages as daiquiris or margaritas, instead choosing 6 ounces of wine. The wine is only 150 calories, versus more than 500 in the margarita. You have worked so hard and love your new body, so keep that foremost in your mind when you decide what to put into that body. If you're going to have a dessert, make it worth your while! The pride you take in your appearance and your health should now filter into everything you put into your body. You deserve the best! So have that decadent brownie, but reduce the portion size, track it, and use it as your only carbohydrate for the meal.

Some tips to help you stay successful:

Meal track: Just because the weight-loss part of your journey is finished doesn't mean meal tracking is over. Meal tracking is and will continue to be a key part of your lifestyle as you move forward, and it's essential for weight maintenance. Not only will meal tracking help you be aware of how many calories you're consuming, it will help keep you accountable for your food intake. Expect to meal track a minimum of three times a week for at least the next two years! The 20/20 LifeStyles online app makes it easy.

Here's a new way to visualize balance: **90/10.** Having one off-plan item every other week is perfectly acceptable, but it can lead you into trouble since one off-plan meal can easily turn into one-off plan day, then two, then a week, and so on.

> *You run into trouble when an off-plan meal turns into an off-plan day, then an off-plan week, and so on.*

Using the 90/10 approach, 90 percent of the time your meal plan is business as usual. This means following your maintenance calorie range and sticking to the lean protein, vegetables, and 1 carbohydrate serving per meal and tracking all your meals and snacks. The other 10 percent refers to the instances where you choose to have a glass of wine with dinner, dessert, or another off-plan item but remember, only one carbohydrate serving per meal. We want you to enjoy these foods, but also to meal track them, limit servings to 300 calories, and enjoy them in moderation. The 90/10 approach is a wonderful way to allow you to indulge in moderation, but also to keep your weight off!

Weigh yourself at least weekly: Weighing yourself is another great way to maintain awareness and accountability with your weight. Consistency is important with weighing, so use the same scale on the same day and same time each week.

Stay active: Exercise is also going to be key for weight maintenance. Finding activities or sports you enjoy can be a great way to burn calories, relieve stress, and have some fun. Don't be afraid to try something new. Try going on a bike ride with your family or friends, or go on a hike.

Exercise is always easier when you enjoy what you are doing. Just as important, too, is continuing to monitor your steps. Using a pedometer daily and aiming for more than 6,000 steps a day can help keep you active through the day when you aren't doing structured exercise.

Have a contingency plan: It's not IF you gain some weight back, it's WHEN. You will gain a few pounds back at some point in your life, and when you do, you need to take action. If you reach your red-light weight, stop and refocus. At this point, make sure you are accurately weighing and measuring your food and meal tracking. If you have reduced your exercise frequency or intensity from your plan, get back into your exercise routine. Seriously consider going back to Stage 2 of the meal plan. We discussed that Stage 2 is your foundation and your safe place. You can return to Stage 2 at any time. Know that maintenance is a lifelong process, and don't be afraid to go back to any previous stage at any time. Be sure you are meal tracking and seriously think about contacting one of our dietitians. There are two ways you can do this. You can use our online application at:

www.2020lifestyles.com/get-started/get-started-online/pricing.aspx

Or, if you live in the Puget Sound area, you can make an appointment to see one of our dietitians or counselors by calling (425) 861-6258 or (877) 559-2020, or by email at 2020lifestyles@proclub.com.

Dining out during maintenance is similar to dining out during Stage 2. In a restaurant, visualize your plate as the plate model-⅓ protein, ⅓ salad and vegetables, and ⅓ carbohydrate. If you order wine, stick to the limit of 1 glass, counting wine as the ONLY carbohydrate for that meal. Normally we recommend not eating grains when dining out but if you do, be extremely cautious when ordering them. We discussed that portions are always too large, and grains are rarely whole grains. If you order a grain, ask for a smaller quantity, portion out ½ cup serving, then double your vegetables and avoid all alcohol. If you find portion control with grains at restaurants is too difficult, avoid them completely.

The danger with overeating carbohydrates is that it can shift your body chemistry back to the point where your hunger and craving return. Once that happens, you risk losing your new body and normal body weight.

EXERCISE FOR LIFE

If you've followed the steps we've outlined, you're exercising at an optimum level for weight maintenance, health, and fitness. You must continue to exercise at this level. However, problems may arise to break your consistency. You'll have illnesses and, possibly, injuries. Life events will divert you temporarily. It's easy to get out of the exercise habit, and any of these diversions can lead to your return to a sedentary lifestyle.

In almost all of these situations, though, you will be able to do some type of exercise. You may not be able to run marathons or climb mountains, but you should be able to walk, swim, or bike. Just because you're unable to do your full workout, don't just do nothing. Do what you're able to do. Do what you can.

When a life event diverts you, try to find out how long the diversion will be. Ask your doctor, boss, or family member when you'll be able to return to normal life activities. Put that date into your phone and PC to remind you to get back to your exercise plan. Remember, if it's been some time since you had a full workout, you must begin slowly. Trying to start at your most strenuous stage will lead to injury and discouragement. The good news is that muscle has memory, and you'll get back into top physical condition much faster than you did initially.

LIFESTYLE FOR LIFE

At this point in your progress, you may be feeling a lot of pride and confidence in what you've accomplished. That's great. It's a powerful feel-good reward that you've earned through all your hard work. But remember, overconfidence is just another form of denial. You are human, and you're programmed to make mistakes. Paradoxically, knowledge of this weakness will make you stronger, while denial can destroy all your good efforts.

In time, all of us forget previous painful experiences, while remembering and even exaggerating the recollection of pleasurable experiences. This natural tendency means that, over time, the misery of limited mobility, limited energy, clothes that don't fit, being out of breath walking up the stairs, and having to take multiple medications for our metabolic disorders will fade. At the same time, the joy of jumping into a pile of French fries, pastries, pancakes, or loaves of fresh bread will intensify. As you can guess, giving in to that tendency won't ever be good for you.

This relapse-transition in thinking is slow and insidious. It creeps up on you through the years. If reading this makes you anxious, that's a good sign. If you're telling yourself, "That's not me, I will NEVER feel that way," you are overconfident.

A little fear about your future success is a good thing and will keep you motivated and vigilant.

294

A technique that has helped many of our alumni maintain their weight is starting Maintainer groups. This is a great way for you to maintain accountability. You and 4-6 others agree to weigh in at a central location on a certain day each week. You have already set a yellow-light number for yourself, and if you're above that number, you have to put one dollar in the kitty. If the next week you're still over, you have to put two dollars in, and if you're not under your yellow-light weight on the third and subsequent weeks, you have to contribute four dollars. Once a year, your group takes the money to do a fun event together. This is a highly motivating, fun way to sustain accountability and support for maintaining your weight.

> *When you feel discouraged-or think you need food to make yourself feel better-refer to your contract and call your support person. Replace your need for food by reminding yourself of the rewards you've achieved through your new lifestyle. This will help refocus you and get you thinking positive, healthy thoughts.*

It's also motivating to keep several pictures of yourself-before and after-on your computer, phone, and bathroom mirror, or even better, on your refrigerator door.

Positive affirmations can also help keep you motivated. Get a stack of 3x5 cards and write a short affirmation on each card. Every morning, right after you get out of bed, read one of the cards. This will help direct your attitude for the whole day. Here are some examples of these affirmations:

- I accept, respect and love myself.

- I am feeling and thinking thin.

- I love feeling healthy.

- I am stronger today than yesterday.

- I have more energy.

- I've been eating and exercising right.

- I'm a more productive and successful person.

- I am improving in every way.

- I'm learning more every day.

- I'm looking good.

- I can look like them, or I can eat like them, but not both.

- It's SO worth it.

- The best way to get back on plan is to not get off it.

- I am just one bite away from gaining 30 pounds.

- I WILL follow my plan today.

- I like the way my clothes fit and look.

- I want to live to see my kids married.

You get the idea, just add your own.

CHAPTER 14

THE NUGGETS- LIFE LESSONS THAT LAST

I CHOSE NOT TO BE A WALKING PHARMACY
Kurt, age 50

It's funny how as life goes by, day after day, you can slide into behavior that you begin to rationalize as acceptable. It's partially denial and partially the fact that the person you've become is simply someone you don't want to deal with just yet-that any looming health issues are something you can put off.

I didn't consider myself an example of fitness or health by any means, but I had accepted who I was physically. I did a bit of exercise, such as playing golf occasionally. I "enjoyed life to the fullest," meaning I never thought about taking care of myself. I ate what I wanted and always put the idea that I might have to change on the back burner.

Well, that back burner was suddenly moved to the front one day 10 years ago as I turned 40. I went to the doctor's office and found myself up to 310 pounds-a weight that was off the charts for a man 6 feet tall.

The doctor's assessment of my health was grim. I was diagnosed as a type 2 diabetic with very high blood pressure, high triglycerides, and high cholesterol. At my weight, the doctor viewed my future as totally predictable. He recommended that I get on medication for all my disorders immediately and forever-meaning I would be on drugs for the rest of my life, and even with the drugs, that might not be for long.

I was stunned. Not that I hadn't accepted the fact that I would someday have to do something about my weight, but hearing the doctor describe my future unless I started taking all those medications was extremely depressing. I was faced with the issue of my own mortality. And this wasn't "someday" any more. It was now or never, and never might mean the end of my life.

Fortunately, something made me skeptical about committing to all the drugs I was told I'd have to take. It may have been instinctive on my part to seek a second opinion, but in this case, the second opinion was my own. As a patient, I simply wasn't ready to succumb to what was considered by many in medicine as the prescribed course of action.

I began to read about statins like Lipitor, blood pressure meds like HCTZ, and of course, the eventuality of insulin injections and all the related health issues brought on by diabetes. What became obvious as I forecast my future was that my life was about to become one large prescription of daily medications, compounded by numerous side effects. Beyond that, even a decade ago, there was some counter thought regarding the long-term use of statins and their side effects, though much of that was discounted as a minor problem-such as a few muscle aches. Today, on the other hand, there's evidence that Lipitor, used long term, can cause breast cancer and diabetes-a disorder I was trying to conquer!

As I was debating what to do back then, a friend recommended I look into 20/20 LifeStyles and their approach to weight loss and curing metabolic disorders.

I went to the introductory seminar given by Dr. Dedomenico and rapidly discovered that 20/20 LifeStyles was far more than a diet. It was a complete lifestyle program supervised by doctors, which included education, exercise, expert advice from registered dietitians, and lifestyle counseling that was meant to change your habits. Doctor Dedomenico's very logical and heartfelt message was so convincing that I turned away from my medicated future and joined 20/20 LifeStyles instead.

That decision saved my life!

You see, because of what I learned from 20/20 LifeStyles, I never took one drug for my metabolic disorders. Not one. And I lost 110 pounds, cured my diabetes, high cholesterol, and high blood pressure, and regained considerable energy and endurance. Rather than stepping onto a merry-go-round of medications that then required other medications to counter their side effects, I totally beat the system.

I know that sounds impossible to some people, who are convinced that medication is the only way to go, but I'm living proof of the alternatives. I am also proud of my physical shape at my age.

After 20/20 LifeStyles guided me through my exercise program, I began to take great joy in hiking and mountain climbing. In fact, a year after I started the 20/20 program, I climbed Mount Rainier, a 14,000-foot mountain in Washington State. I've climbed it twice since then, plus mountains in South America and Gannett Peak in Wyoming. If I may say so, I've become an exceptional climber and hiker-not bad for a guy who used to have trouble climbing a flight of stairs.

If I can leave you with one thought, it's this: Health is a matter of choice. You have it in your power to choose the right lifestyle and the right state of mind.

At 20/20 LifeStyles, that state of mind has been described as the self-slimming mindset. It works because it begins with the self-in other words, you. You have the final responsibility for your health. The sooner you come to that realization, the quicker you can make your life a tribute to wellbeing. If you haven't taken responsibility for your health and life yet, I encourage you to be like me and do it. Not tomorrow but today.

Kurt recently returned from a climb up Mount Everest-from 310-pound couch potato to world-class mountain climber! This amazing transformation could only happen because he learned and lived the lessons listed in this chapter.

Don't forget, we want to hear your stories too. Send us your stories, successes, and challenges. Send them to lifestylesbook@proclub.com.

THE KEY TAKEAWAYS TO THE SELF-SLIMMING MINDSET

While this book contains a tremendous amount of valuable information, we realize that your mind can only absorb a limited amount of material at one time. That's why we advise you to use this book as a reference source. Go back and read over sections when you find yourself having problems, or if you just want to refer back to information on a particular topic. Be sure to look at the appendixes, which contain recipes, information, and other aids for your 20/20 LifeStyles plan.

In this chapter, we hope to assist you in keeping your focus by giving you The Nuggets, 31 gems of information absolutely essential to have if you want to maintain your new health, body, and mind for the rest of your life.

Nugget #1: Self-acceptance, self-respect, and self-love are essential for positive self-change.

You have to start with self-acceptance, which means you **MUST** get rid of the guilt and shame. In order to help rid you of these destructive feelings we discussed how your overweight and metabolic issues were not your fault. Remember, the majority of Americans are in the same boat as you, and for the same reasons. Your nutritional education has been faulty, many of the foods available to you were unhealthy, and the food industry has a huge interest in persuading you to eat more and more inexpensive foods made from sugar, fat, salt, and high-fructose corn syrup. Many of those foods are grain based and high in sugar, others are liquids rich in high-fructose corn syrup. So as you can see, it's not your fault(32).

Nugget #2: Replacing love with food will cause you to feel unloved and depressed.

Our culture often confuses food with love. As a little boy or girl, when you skinned your knee, your mother gave you a cookie. On a special date, birthday, or anniversary you were taken out to a nice restaurant and consumed a meal high in sugar, fat, and salt. As you gained weight and felt more unlovable, you tried to correct that by eating more food to stimulate your reward center, which just made you feel even more unlovable. The answer to dealing with this syndrome is found in self-respect and self-love. Treating your body with respect will make you feel more lovable, because doing so is a true form of self-love, and unlike the food-for-love cycle, it makes you feel better, not worse

Nugget #3: It is easy to let your lapses move you back to self-blame and guilt.

If you allow self-blame to creep back into your thinking, you block your path to progress. You must remember that you are human, and as such, you will sometimes fail. Instead of beating yourself up for your failures, you must analyze them, without blame, and try to learn from them, so that you can avoid them in the future as we discussed in Chapter 12.

32. *See video Intro Seminar 1 under Free Videos in Appendix J.*

Nugget #4: Hopelessness is just another symptom of a closed mind.

When you wall yourself off from any input that may be able to help your situation, you negate the possibility of change. Hopelessness can manifest itself in many ways: "I can't do this," "I tried it and it didn't work," "This is too hard," "These things never work for me," "I'm not the same as those others who succeed," etc. Hopelessness is your own personal prison, and since it is your own prison, you have the key. *The key is not allowing your fear of failure to keep you from trying.* Remember, you're only a failure when you stop trying to succeed.

Nugget #5: What you think of yourself is far more important than what others think of you.

Public opinion is very fickle, and today's hero often winds up being tomorrow's villain. If you have self-acceptance, self-respect, and self-love, you will find that others will accept, respect, and love you.

Nugget #6: When your body is out of balance, it is very difficult to eat, exercise, and think right.

Getting on track, or back on track, can be difficult. But remember, the hardest part is starting, after that it gets much easier. The withdrawal from a carbohydrate-rich diet rarely lasts more than 3 days. You can do that!

The diet that Americans eat was **NOT** designed for the genetic makeup of your body. As human bodies evolve, we are not very distant from our hunter-gatherer ancestors. And yet we eat more sugar and other carbohydrates in a day than our ancestors ate in a year, and it's killing us. Our hunter-gatherer ancestors ate mainly nuts, vegetables, fruits, and occasional lean meats. All meats were lean, because there were no farm animals, only wild animals, and it was difficult for our ancestors to catch and kill these animals without winding up on the menu themselves.

Nugget #7: Support is essential to maintain a healthy lifestyle.

Sometimes that support can come from family or friends, but there are times when you have to reach out and develop new support systems. This can be challenging. In childhood, most of us make new friends easily. A new kid moves into the neighborhood, and we're playing with him or her the next day. In adult life, it seems to be much more difficult. We feel shy and awkward. We think we may be rejected. Once again, fear is our enemy, and we must break through that fear. Remember, MOST NORMAL-WEIGHTED PEOPLE DON'T UNDERSTAND YOU. It's important to have at least one or two support people who understand your metabolic disorder. And, don't forget, support, not food, is an honest way to show love. If you're having difficulty finding support, see Appendix A for ways you can get support from 2020lifestyles.com.

Nugget #8: Assertiveness is a necessary component of a healthy lifestyle.

Codependents, who always place others first, lack this ability. Placing yourself first and being able to say "No" are foundations for self-acceptance, self-respect, and self-love. Clearly, if you feel you are not important enough to place your wellbeing above all else, you cannot achieve health or happiness. And if you aren't healthy or happy, you become part of the problem rather than part of the solution, so in fact you're helping nobody.

Nugget #9: Your diet may be destroying your brain.

Many of you take as much or more pride in your mind than you do in your body. But your unhealthy and destructive consumption of foods high in sugar, fat, refined grains, and nonnatural sugars are slowly damaging your brains. Because the process is slow, and because it affects your mind, it's hard to detect until it's too late. Most of you have known someone who has dementia or Alzheimer's disease. You knew them when they were bright, functional individuals, and you're saddened and disturbed when you see what has happened to their minds. Make no mistake, the damage that unhealthy eating causes to your brain is every bit as destructive as the damage it does to your health and lifestyle.

Nugget #10: One of the most important tools for your healthy lifestyle is meal tracking.

We can't overemphasize the importance of this tool. First and foremost, tracking within 15 minutes of eating is a behavior and habit-change intervention. JUST TRACKING WHAT YOU EAT WILL CHANGE WHAT YOU EAT! What a painless way to change your eating habits! Additionally, meal tracking will teach you how to analyze your reactions to various foods, about your body chemistry, and how your diet affects your body. In addition to recording what you eat, you also need to record your reactions to foods. If you experience heartburn, bloating, or other unpleasant symptoms when you eat certain foods, meal tracking helps you make the connection so you can omit them from your diet. Most importantly, meal tracking helps you know what foods cause you to experience hunger or craving. Lastly, meal tracking will help you keep focus on what you are doing and why you are doing it [33].

Nugget #11: Keep the junk food out of the house, car, office, etc.

Sometimes all it takes is a few minutes for rationality to return. If the junk food isn't in the house, car, or office, its absence gives you some thinking time. Give yourself that time by not having the unhealthy foods within easy reach.

---

33. See *Self-Monitoring for Success in Lifestyle Series* in Appendix J.

Nugget #12: Exercise, non-exercise activity (NEAT), adequate sleep, and stress management are all part of a healthy lifestyle.

The rationalizations for not exercising are voluminous, but sometimes you just need to go on autopilot, shut off your brain, and get your workout clothes on. In other words, "Just do it." NEAT is also very important in maintaining a healthy weight. It's almost impossible to compensate for inadequate NEAT with exercise, because NEAT occurs during all your waking hours. You must use your pedometer at least 3-4 days per week. Some individuals use it every day for life. Without adequate sleep, your body gets out of chemical balance. You begin to crave sweets and other carbohydrates, and your hunger increases. Stress, depression, and sleep deprivation cause your body to produce increased levels of cortisol and put you into insulin resistance. That causes increased hunger and increased fat storage.

Nugget #13: Foods rich in sugar, fat, and salt stimulate the reward center (pleasure center) of the brain.

They also increase the production of the feel-good chemicals: serotonin, beta-endorphin, and dopamine. Serotonin, as most of you know, makes you feel happier; endorphins make you feel relaxed and relieve all those little aches and pains. But the real problem is dopamine. Dopamine intensifies your focus, and when that focus is on a food rich in sugar, fat, and salt, that intensified focus is called a craving. What's worse, the more often you eat these foods, the stronger the cravings become.

And don't forget that many of the foods labeled "diet," "light," "low fat," or "sugar free" can be unhealthy and loaded with calories. You must get into the habit of reading labels and remember that almost always, food ingredients ending in "ose" are some form of sugar. Lastly, if you can't identify an ingredient, don't eat it!

Nugget #14: Alcohol is the diet destroyer.

Alcohol signals your body to store energy (fat and sugar) instead of burning it. This stops weight loss. Additionally, alcohol is dead calories-that is, it contains no nutritional value. And lastly, alcohol is a disinhibitor, which means it negatively affects your judgment, which can lead to unhealthy eating.

Nugget #15: Dining out can be a challenge.

Don't open the restaurant menu unless you really have to. Order what you want, specify the quantities you need, and say you want no extra sauces, butter, or oils on your foods. Remember, the plate is ⅓ protein, ⅓ salad or vegetables, and ⅓ carbohydrate, and an alcoholic beverage substitutes for the entire carbohydrate portion of your plate. It's also best to stay away from all grains when eating out.

Nugget #16: The stages of change are pre-contemplation, contemplation, preparation, action, and maintenance.

Remember, denial, rationalization, or minimization can take you from maintenance right back into pre-contemplation. You must always be on guard when you hear yourself starting to justify unhealthy eating, not exercising, not sleeping, or lapsing back into negative thinking.

Nugget #17: Protein and vegetables will be the mainstay of your food plan for life.

If you find yourself drifting back into unhealthy eating patterns, Stage 2 is the road back to controlling your diet and your health. A week on Stage 2 removes the chemical pull that causes you to eat unhealthy foods or unhealthy amounts of food, allowing your body to get back into balance.

Nugget #18: Unhealthy foods are both the reward and the punishment.

These foods rapidly stimulate the feel-good chemicals in your brain but later cause you to be very unhappy about your weight and your health. In behavioral terms, the reward is much more powerful than the punishment because of the time factor. The reward happens almost immediately, while the punishment comes much later.

Nugget #19: Binge eaters must beware of old habits.

Those of you who are binge eaters should be aware of just how fast you can gain weight, or gain back the weight you've lost. If the criteria we discussed in Chapter 4, Concept #15, apply to you, then you must follow certain steps. If you find yourself hiding your eating, eating after dinner, not exercising, and not being honest with your support people, then you're in trouble. You must find help, and find it quickly. Talk to a psychologist or counselor in your area with experience in treating binge-eating disorder. Remember, DO NOT DELAY, because your eating disorder can make you gain weight very rapidly, and if you've been diligent with the 20/20 LifeStyles plan up to that point, it would be a pity to undo all your good work in a short time.

Nugget #20: The fastest way back to your old unhealthy lifestyle is to lose control of your time.

That's extremely easy to do, because lifestyle has gravity. By that, we mean it wants to pull you back. Your kids still want 120 percent of your time, your significant other insists on having time, your boss still wants you to work 60 hours per week, you still spend hours surfing the internet and playing online games, and if you say "No" to your friends too often, they stop calling. The demands and the pressures haven't changed, but you've made the hard choices and forced yourself and those around you to respect your time plan. That requires a lot of energy, and you'll need to keep spending that energy.

Nugget #21: Accept yourself, respect yourself, love yourself, and respect your body.

That means keeping your body in chemical balance-and a very delicate balance that is. Your body has a complex system of chemical and nerve communications that try to keep you in balance, but if you push it too far, you override all the systems that try to protect you. The result is a chemical chain reaction that leads you to illness, disability, and early death. The best way to show yourself love is to help your body help you, not destroy it with the wrong kinds and amounts of food.

Nugget #22: Diabetes is a slow and very unpleasant way to die.

As of 2011, there were 106 million people in this country with diabetes or pre-diabetes. Like Kurt, you could be one of them, or you could be on your way to becoming one. But 97 percent of the diabetes in this country is type 2. That means IT IS PREVENTABLE! If you follow the 20/20 LifeStyles plan, the probability of your developing this deadly disease is dramatically reduced. If you have type 2 diabetes and follow this plan, the probability dramatically increases that you'll eventually be able to discontinue your medications, have a normal blood sugar, and lead a healthy life. Just ask Kurt about that.

Simple carbohydrates start turning to sugar in your mouth before they even reach your stomach, so they count as sugar in our meal plan. As we discussed, eating foods rich in sugars or simple carbohydrates causes a rapid spike in your blood-sugar levels, followed by a corresponding crash in those blood-sugar levels about 60-90 minutes later. This rapid decrease in blood-sugar levels causes you to seek more high-sugar and carbohydrate foods. Foods high in protein, however, cause a much more gradual rise in your blood-sugar levels, and those levels also decline much more slowly. Limiting your carbohydrate intake to 1 portion per meal and always eating a lean protein, or a very lean protein with a heart-healthy fat serving, as part of every meal and snack will protect you from that blood-sugar crash.

Nugget #23: Habits are set in very "low" levels of the brain.

Habits are almost automatic, and therefore very difficult to change. They're so automatic that often you're completely unaware of them. Therefore, the first step in changing habits is to make yourself aware of them and aware of the things that cue or trigger the habits. Keeping a log or diary is a very good way to increase that awareness. Once you're aware of your unhealthy habits, you can start to change them. You can modify these habits by avoiding the cueing environments, and by changing your keystone habits. Changing keystone habits will start a cascade of habit change. The good news is that you are now creating new habits, but remember, it takes up to 2-3 years for these new habits to become fixed.

Nugget #24: In order to develop the self-slimming mindset you must gain control of your self-talk.

If you're constantly berating yourself, criticizing yourself, and putting yourself down, you can't improve. If you're telling yourself that you will fail, that there's no hope, and that this is way too hard for you, you will fail. You must modify your self-talk so that it passes the truth test. The truth test means that it is logical, rational, and not simply based on your emotional state of the moment.

Nugget #25: Visualization is a powerful tool to help you change your behavior. You can use it to get through difficult situations more easily. You can use it to help overcome the fear of making changes, and you can also use it to see yourself being slim, healthy, and happy. Visualization is a first step in preparing yourself to become the new you.

Nugget #26: Your body's appetite-regulation system works by both releasing chemicals and directly stimulating nerves to signal hunger or satiety.

Chemical signaling is fairly slow and takes up to 20 minutes to inform your brain that you're no longer hungry. In order to allow that process to occur normally, you must use mindful eating techniques. And mindful eating relies on other factors we've mentioned, such as time management. Clearly, you can't take the time to eat in a mindful way if your time is out of control and you're eating on the run. Mindful eating requires you to focus on your food, pause between bites, and eat slowly, giving your body a chance to register the effects of the food you have eaten.

Nugget #27: Good health means being different.

Unfortunately, in our society, if you want to lead a healthy lifestyle, you have to be a nonconformist. When ⅔ of the population is overweight, by definition, those who chose to achieve normal weight are in the minority. Resisting social pressures, food industry advertising, and pressure from friends, family, and business associates is not easy. You must leave the pack, and you must have a clear vision of why doing so is necessary for you.

Nugget #28: We can't overstate the damage sugar can do.

Americans eat too much sugar, and it's destroying their lives and killing them at an early age. Here are some things sugars-and, remember carbohydrates are sugars-cause:

- Visceral adiposity, that very dangerous buildup of fat in your abdomen that leads to metabolic syndrome, heart disease, stroke, cancer, etc.

- Suppression of your immune system

- Increased inflammatory response in your entire body

- A rise in the levels of fat circulating in your blood, leading to atherosclerosis (hardening of the arteries)

- Damage to your kidneys and liver

- Damage to your arteries and heart

- Stomach problems

- Vision problems

- And many more health problems.

Always read the labels on food, and remember that ingredients ending in "ose" are almost always sugars. Avoid them!

Nugget #29: Be constantly aware of lapses and relapses.

In order not to slowly lapse back into unhealthy eating and living, you must work to keep a top-of-mind awareness of what you are doing and why you are doing it. In order to do this, you must have a support system that includes others like you: friends and workout buddies. Additionally, you need to be involved in sports activities and activities that continually help you focus on the benefits of your new life and health: such things as helping others to health, having "Before" pictures of yourself where you will see them each day and yes, MEAL TRACKING.

A lapse is when you allow your eating, exercise, and lifestyle to get out of control for a short time period. A relapse is a prolonged episode of lack of control that leads you to regain either a substantial portion or all the weight you lost. Lapses will happen because you are human, and you cannot maintain perfection indefinitely. The key is to recognize a lapse early on and take action, thereby preventing a relapse. The first thing you need to do is forgive yourself. Remember self-acceptance? You need the feelings of self-respect and self-love to put you back on track to respecting your body. The second step is to analyze what went wrong. That way it becomes a learning experience and will be preventable in the future. Next, create a plan for dealing with similar situations and rehearse that plan using visualization.

Nugget #30: To prevent relapse, keep the motivation alive.

When you first lose a substantial amount of weight on the 20/20 LifeStyles plan, life is great! Everyone is complimenting you on how good you look; you fit into your smaller-sized, more fashionable clothes; you're enjoying physical activity; and you feel healthy every day. The newness of this experience is quite powerful, but unfortunately newness doesn't last forever. After some time, no one tells you how great it is that you haven't changed your appearance. The clothes still fit the same, you're used to your physical capabilities, and you feel normal. The thrill is gone, and often the motivation goes with it. In order to prevent that from happening, you have to spend some time and energy keeping that motivation alive. If you don't, you WILL relapse. On a regular basis, dig out the contract you wrote to yourself and review the following:

- Are you weighing yourself regularly?

- Are you responding to yellow- and red-light weights as you agreed?

- Are you working out at the intensity, frequency, and regularity you agreed to?

- Are you wearing your pedometer and keeping track of your NEAT?

- Are you staying in contact with your support people and workout buddies?

- Are you using visualization to help you through tough times and keep you motivated?

- Are you staying on top of your time management and saying "No" when you need to?

ARE YOU MEAL TRACKING?

If you aren't doing these things, you ARE losing motivation and will eventually relapse.

Nugget #31: This book was written for you!

You are a human being, one who wrestled with weight for a long time and had been defeated. This book is designed to help you turn that defeat, depression, and hopelessness into victory, joy, and health. This book is not designed for the person trying their first weight-loss diet. That person hasn't experienced the pain you have; that person still believes that losing weight and keeping it off will be easy. You know better, and because of that, you may be willing to follow the path so carefully outlined in the 20/20 LifeStyles plan.

Our approach is not a hypothetical model or test; it has worked for over 10,000 people just like you. Our hope is that one or all of the personal stories told in this book by 20/20 program participants were stories that spoke to you. These 10 stories are only a small sampling of the 10,000 people we've helped, and yet all of those 10,000 stories would display the same basic characteristics. Those 10,000 stories would illustrate how the men and women telling them failed at diets and hated themselves for failing. They would show how, despite illnesses and feeling sick every day, they continued to eat unhealthy foods and gain weight. They didn't want to be that way, but they just couldn't effect any lasting change. Those 10,000 stories would repeatedly demonstrate how people who were beaten latched onto the same concepts we've given you in these pages and became happy and healthy individuals.

On the other hand, those 10,000 stories would not be told by people who thought the process was easy, or that once they lost the weight they could return to their old habits and lifestyles. On the contrary, they would be told by people who were desperate enough to fight one more time, and to invest the time and effort necessary for success.

Just as you can identify with their pain, you can also identify with their perseverance and with their success. You can write your own story, and it can be the best story of them all.

APPENDIX
RESOURCES FOR HEALTH

APPENDIX A

SERVICES AVAILABLE AT 2020LIFESTYLES.COM

Many services available at 2020lifestyles.com can help you with your food plan and your new life. These services will be familiar to you and will fit in well with the material you have read in 20/20 LifeStyles. Take some time to explore this website and see how much interesting and helpful material is available to you there.

If you're having problems or just want to speed up your weight loss, you may want to consider purchasing a monthly package that includes more support and online tools. Here are some of the packages available to you:

- **Essentials:** Get started for FREE and bring your health back into balance. Get instant access to our online tools and Stages 1 and 2 content packs, including meal plans, cooking videos, workout videos, nutrition guides, and recipes.

- **Essentials Plus:** This great package provides you with access to content packs for all 7 stages, including meal plans, cooking videos, workout videos, nutrition guides, and recipes, as well as our Ask An Expert Service and Weekly Dietitian Review service. This package also includes our delicious Sample Product Kit.

- **Ask an Expert:** Access to your own personal dietitian or personal trainer at your fingertips. These services allows you to ask our experts questions about your meal plan, your exercise routine, and building healthy lifestyle habits. You will receive a response within 5 minutes. Your support team is just one click away!

- **Weekly Dietitian Review:** This service allows you and your dietitian to work together via your Health Tracker. By tracking your daily food choices, water intake, exercise pattern, etc., your dietitian will be able to provide you with personalized advice and guidance for how best to achieve your nutrition and health goals. Your dietitian will help you develop a food routine for successful weight loss and weight maintenance.

- **Premium Package:** Lose weight and keep it off with everything you need to succeed. A monthly package allowing complete access to Stages 1-7 content packs, Ask An Expert, Weekly Dietitian Review, and a monthly shipment of 20/20 LifeStyles nutritional products for your meal plan.

APPENDIX B

GHRELIN - THE HUNGER HORMONE

The body has two routes for sending messages: the nervous system and the endocrine system. The nervous system sends messages almost immediately. If you place your hand on a hot stove, a message is sent to your brain telling you that your hand is in pain and should be removed immediately. Communication through the endocrine system is significantly slower. The endocrine system communicates using chemicals secreted from glands or organs in your body. These chemicals can originate in your stomach, pancreas, or many other organs or glands and will eventually enter the bloodstream.

These chemicals circulate through your entire body, but certain locations in your body contain specific receptors that allow only specific chemicals to enter. When that specific chemical begins to enter the receptor, the receptor sends a message to your body to respond in a certain way. These chemicals that travel through the blood are called hormones.

One of the hormones bodies produce is called ghrelin. It's produced in the stomach, when the stomach is empty. It enters the bloodstream, and when it reaches its receptor site in the brain, it tells your brain you're hungry and need to find food (Figure 1.01).

Figure 1.01

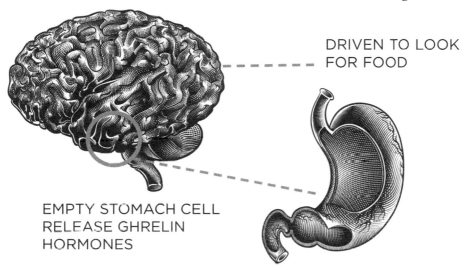

DRIVEN TO LOOK
FOR FOOD

EMPTY STOMACH CELL
RELEASE GHRELIN
HORMONES

This is the explanation for the basic hunger drive we all have. When the stomach is empty, it sends a message to the brain saying, "Find food!" This is one hormone we can and need to control. Figure 1.02 shows how ghrelin levels vary throughout the day.

Figure 1.02

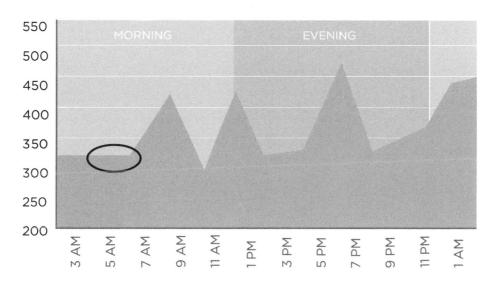

If you were to wake up at 3:00 in the morning, your stomach would have been empty for 6 to 8 hours, but you aren't hungry. As you can see, even though you haven't eaten for some time, your ghrelin levels are quite low. That's because there's an overriding system that governs ghrelin production in our body, called circadian rhythm.

If you regularly go to bed at 11:00 p.m. and wake at 7:00 a.m., you may not even need an alarm clock, because your body knows this is your normal rhythm. Therefore, even though your stomach is empty at 11:00 p.m., your body knows you're in your sleep cycle, so it will stop your stomach from producing ghrelin.

If you happen to work night shifts and then try to live on a day schedule on days when you are not working nights, you'll distort your circadian rhythm and gain weight easily. But there's a way of correcting that problem. Working with a number of people who have that issue, we have them exercise at the same time of day or night, regardless of whether they're in their day-sleeping or night-sleeping cycle. We usually have them exercise in the afternoon between 3:00 p.m. and 5:00 p.m. This returns them to normal circadian rhythm. Figure 1.03 shows a normal ghrelin cycle for a person who gets up at 6:45 a.m.

Figure 1.03

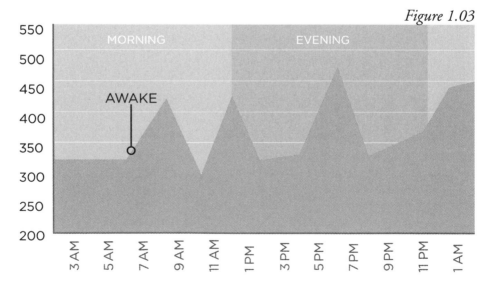

Your body's circadian rhythm knows that you're going to wake at 6:45 a.m., so it starts producing ghrelin around 5:00 a.m. You wake mildly hungry and have breakfast. As soon as food enters your stomach, ghrelin production stops, and the blood level of ghrelin begins to drop until your stomach is empty (around 10:00 a.m.), at which point your stomach will start producing ghrelin again (Figure 1.04).

Figure 1.04

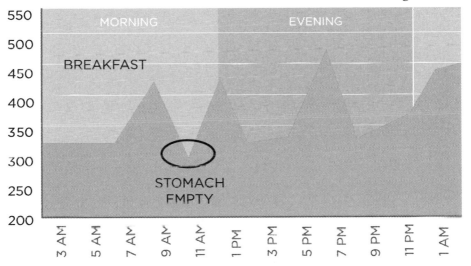

The ghrelin level continues to increase until 12:00 p.m. (lunch time). Again, you'll find yourself mildly hungry, but once you eat, the ghrelin level decreases again until your stomach is empty (Figure 1.05).

Figure 1.05

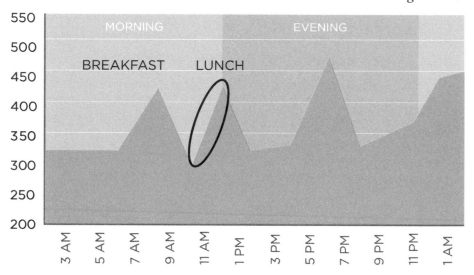

Usually at breakfast and lunch you don't feel like you're starving. However, look what happens between lunch and dinner (Figure 1.06).

Figure 1.06

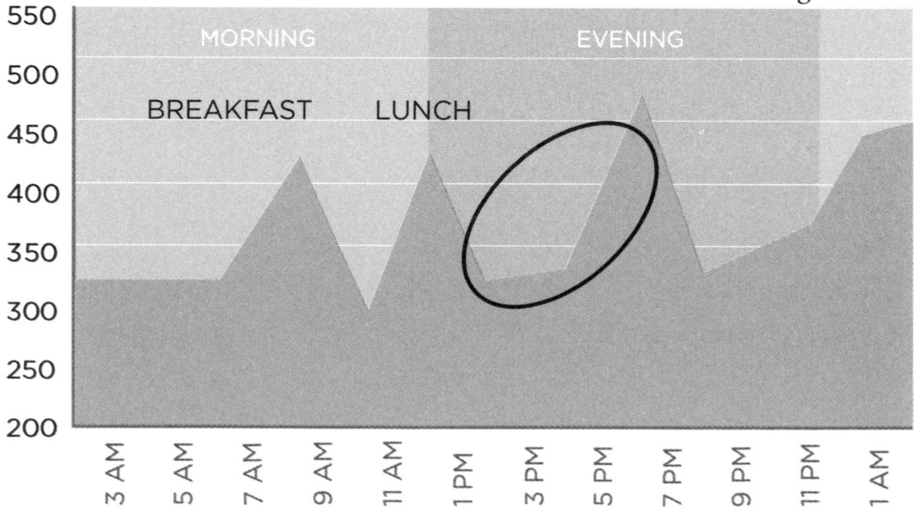

Ghrelin levels decrease until your stomach is empty (about 2:00 p.m.) and then begin rising. Because of the longer time between lunch and dinner (usually 6-7 hours), by dinner time your ghrelin level is the highest of the day (Figure 1.07).

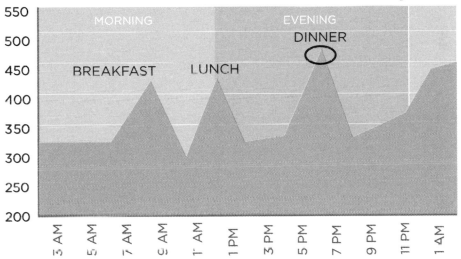

Figure 1.07

So the problem will be regulating your dinner meal. Suppose you go to your favorite restaurant for dinner, and when the waitress asks if you want something to drink, you say "Yes, I'd like a glass of wine." Then she slides the nice warm loaf of bread onto the table, and you eat the whole loaf. Afterward, she comes back with the wine and replenishes the bread. And when your significant other says, "You're going to wreck your dinner," now you can say, "Honey, my ghrelin level is so high I can't help it. I'm being driven by my ghrelin." And you're right. However, once you eat dinner, the ghrelin level drops (Figure 1.08).

Figure 1.08

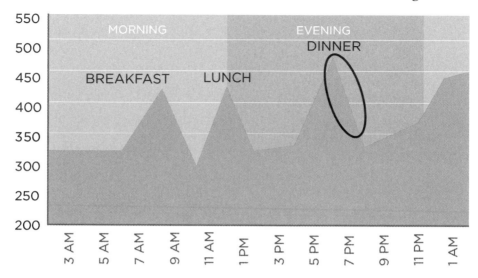

If you go to bed around 9:00 or 10:00 p.m. you're okay, your ghrelin level is manageable, and your circadian rhythm will cause your ghrelin blood level to drop (Figure 1.09).

Figure 1.09

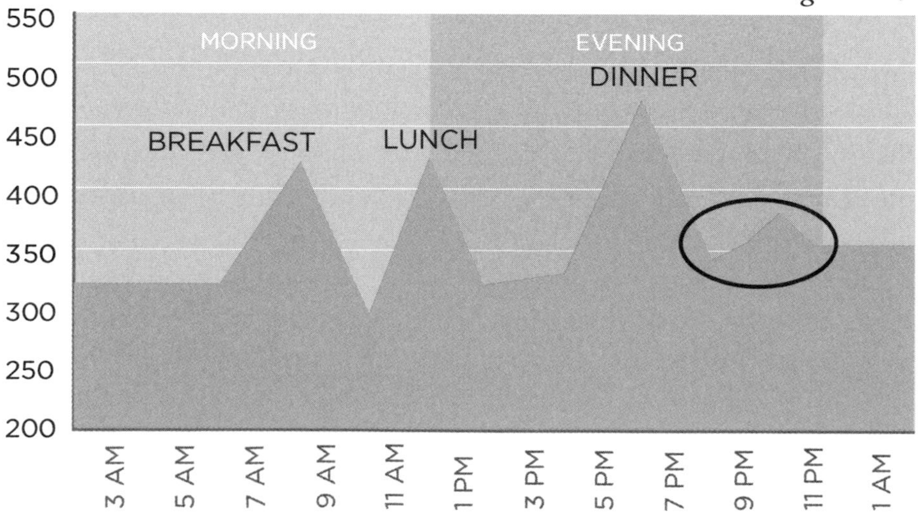

If you stay up playing Xbox or working on your computer, you can see how your ghrelin gets higher than at breakfast or lunch (Figure 1.10).

Figure 1.10

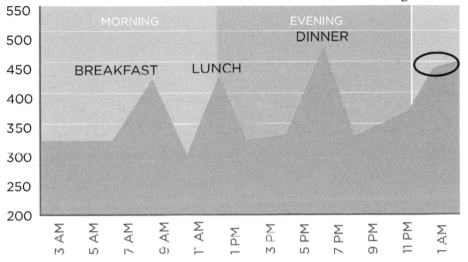

Because your ghrelin level is so high, not only do you experience hunger, you tend to lose control of your eating, so you head for the kitchen to eat whatever you can find.

Ghrelin production is, however, relatively easy to control. Anytime you'll have longer than 4 hours between meals, you'll need a snack. You'll notice that the preceding graphics only show about 4 hours between breakfast and lunch. But if you happen to have an early breakfast and more than 4 hours elapses between breakfast and lunch, then you should add a snack to control your ghrelin. Using our graphic, with an obvious span of more than 4 hours between lunch and dinner, you'd need a snack during that period. Figure 1.11 demonstrates how the snack affects your ghrelin level.

Figure 1.11

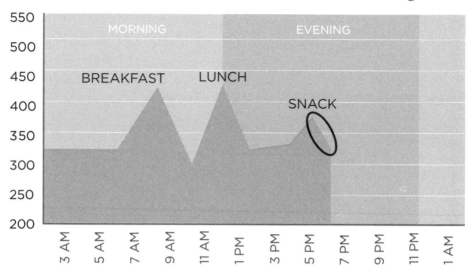

The snack entering your stomach causes your ghrelin level to decrease, making it much easier to manage your hunger at dinnertime. The same applies if you're going to stay up late. Have a snack at about 9:00 p.m., so your ghrelin drops again (Figure 1.12). That way, you won't get out-of-control hungry at night.

Figure 1.12

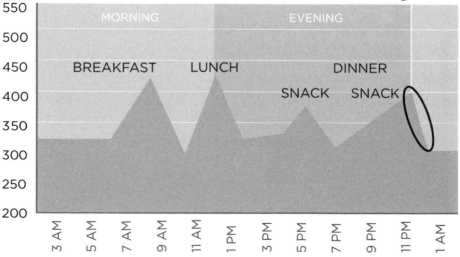

At the time when you should be eating your afternoon and evening snacks, you probably won't feel hungry. Remember, you're eating the snacks so you don't get hungry later. By eating 3 meals plus 1-2 snacks, you're able to manage your ghrelin levels and control your hunger.

If you don't eat breakfast, your ghrelin levels will continue to rise, and you'll be extremely hungry at lunchtime, so you'll overeat (Figure 1.13).

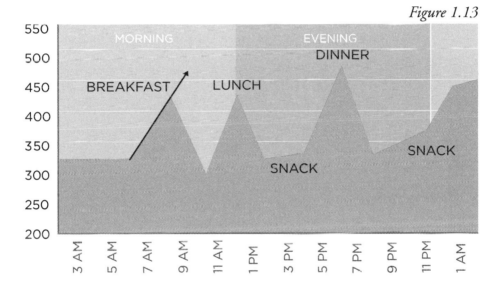

Figure 1.13

Controlling your production of ghrelin also causes your metabolism to increase, which helps you burn more calories. Also, if you have your evening meal or snack and then don't eat again for 10-12 hours each day, the 10-hour fast until breakfast will further raise your metabolism and increase your calorie burn.

Now you understand why eating 3 meals and 1-2 snacks per day helps you control your hunger and increase your metabolism.

APPENDIX C

REVERSING LEPTIN RESISTANCE AND INSULIN RESISTANCE WITH EXERCISE

Leptin is a hormone that is manufactured in your fat cells. It travels though the bloodstream to receptors in the brain.

Figure 2.01

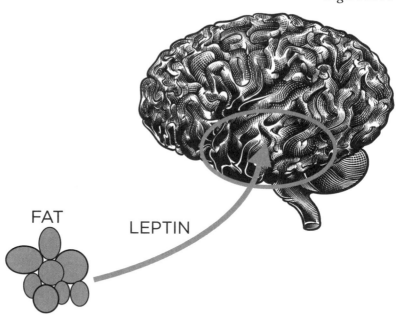

FAT

LEPTIN

Leptin is a long-term regulator of food intake. It's also an appetite suppressant, so if you have more or larger fat cells, you'll produce more leptin. This is called maintaining your set-point weight. Overeating causes your fat cells to increase in size and produce more leptin, which reduces your appetite. Loss of weight reduces leptin production and makes you hungry.

However, there's a problem with this seemingly sophisticated weight-maintenance system. People who are overweight produce leptin, but their brain receptor sites don't respond to leptin. Something blocks the leptin receptors in the brain, keeping the leptin from reaching the receptors. As a result, long-term food regulation fails, and in the end you gain weight.

Scientists have isolated three proteins produced by your body that block the leptin receptor sites and keep the leptin from making its attachment. This condition, called leptin resistance, can be caused by four conditions.

The first condition is being overweight. When you're overweight, you produce these proteins. So, weight-gain blocks the function of leptin; in other words, being overweight blocks our long-term food regulation.

A second condition that will cause leptin resistance is a high-fat diet. Eating a high-fat diet will certainly cause you to lose your long-term ability to regulate food intake.

A third condition that causes leptin blockage or leptin resistance is elevated blood sugar. You need not be diabetic for this condition to arise; all you need is a higher than normal blood sugar, known as hyperglycemia. You become hyperglycemic by eating large amounts of sugars and simple carbohydrates.

And fourth, these proteins are also released by having high blood-insulin levels, or hyperinsulinemia. Insulin is a hormone secreted into the blood by the pancreas, its job being to cause sugar or glucose from the bloodstream into the body's cells. Many overweight and sedentary people have hyperinsulinemia (high levels of insulin in the blood). Their insulin level rises because it's trying to drive the blood sugar into the body's cells. Overweight and obese people who don't exercise were found in our study to have hyperinsulinemia or high levels of insulin in their blood about 90 percent of the time. This is also called insulin resistance, because the insulin isn't effective at causing sugar to enter your cells.

Figure 2.02

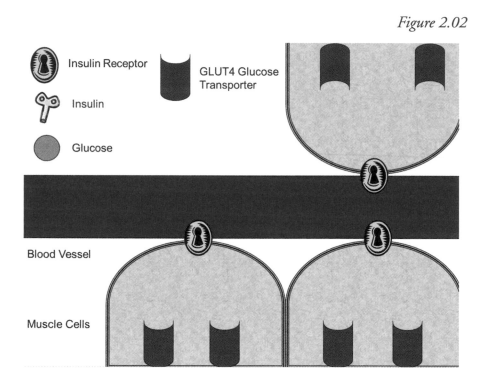

Figure 2.02 represents three little muscle cells and a tiny blood vessel going past them. In this graphic, we've shown one insulin-receptor site on each of the muscle cells, although in actuality there are many more. In a normally functioning cell, the glucose transporters come to the surface of the cell when they are prompted to do so by insulin, and they pick up the sugar and transport it into the cell.

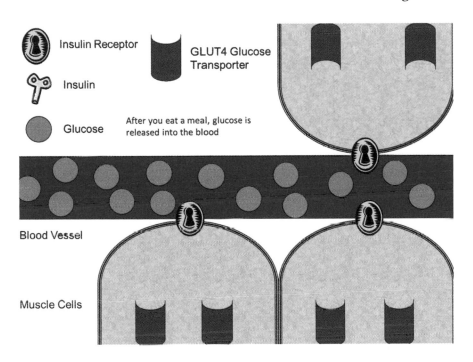

Figure 2.03

After a meal, the sugar or glucose in your blood increases (Fig. 2.03), signaling your pancreas to begin releasing insulin to help move sugar into the cells. The circulating insulin attaches to the receptors (Fig. 2.04), which causes several chemical reactions inside the cells and tells the glucose transporters to move to the surface of the cell (Fig 2.05).

Figure 2.04

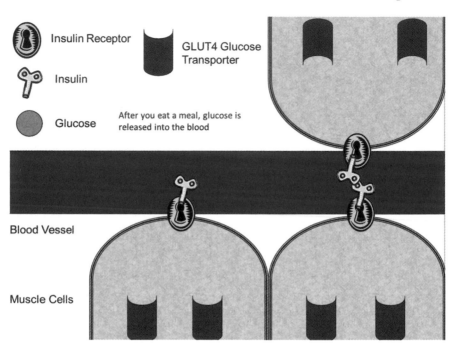

Insulin Receptor

GLUT4 Glucose Transporter

Insulin

Glucose

After you eat a meal, glucose is released into the blood

Blood Vessel

Muscle Cells

Figure 2.05

Insulin Receptor

GLUT4 Glucose Transporter

Insulin

Glucose binds to the transporters and are taken back into the cell

Glucose

Blood Vessel

Muscle Cells

Sugar in the blood gets bound to those transporters and is taken into the cells where it is immediately used for energy or is stored for later use (Figure 2.05).

That's how this system should work. However, if you have insulin resistance, you're not able to bring the sugar into your cells as quickly as needed. Our theory on insulin resistance is that there's too much fat circulating through the body, and too much fat gets into your cells. This excess fat blocks the signal from the insulin receptor, which normally tells the transporters to come to the surface and pick up the sugar. Figure 2.06 illustrates this.

Figure 2.06

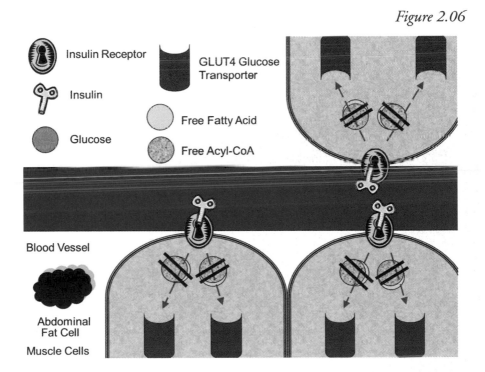

Since the level of your blood sugar remains high, the pancreas continues to release more insulin trying to drive the sugar into the cells. The result of this excessive insulin release, coupled with poor sugar uptake by your cells, causes hyperinsulinemia and hyperglycemia (Fig. 2.07). These are the two factors that cause the body to release the proteins that cause leptin resistance.

So, your blood sugar rises from eating, and your insulin reaches its receptor site. The insulin starts the chemical reaction, but the fat in the cells blocks the chemical reaction from signaling the glucose transporter to rise to the surface of the cell. Your blood sugar stays at the higher level, and the pancreas reacts to the unchanged blood-sugar level by releasing more and more insulin into the blood, trying to drive the sugar into the cells. The end result is a high level of circulating insulin in the blood, or hyperinsulinemia (Figure 2.07).

Figure 2.07

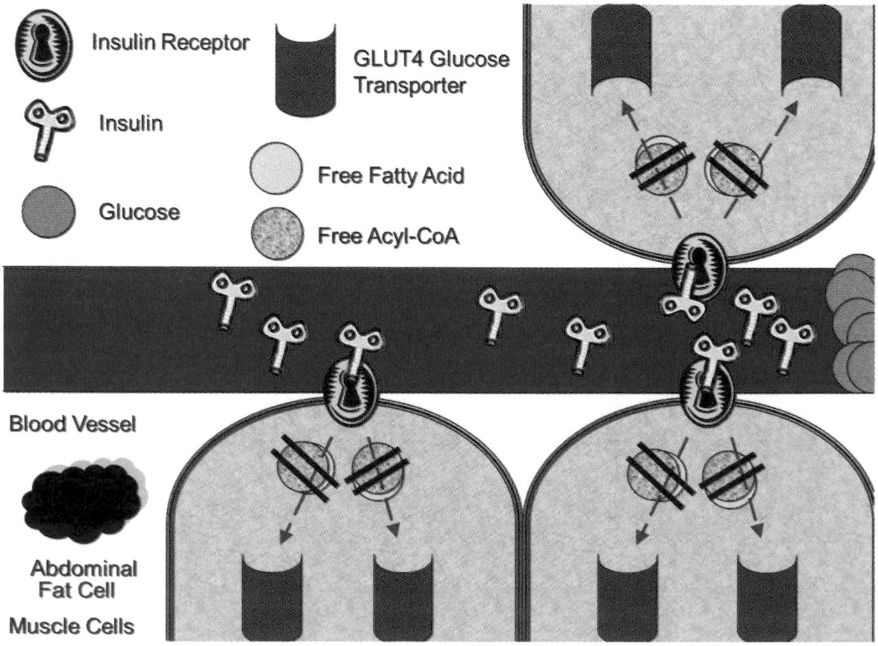

Eventually, sugar will enter the cells, yet you may still have a higher than normal level of sugar (glucose) in your blood, called hyperglycemia. So, when you have insulin resistance, your insulin isn't functioning as it should, and in addition to that state of hyperinsulinemia, you can also have hyperglycemia; both are conditions that cause leptin resistance. In practical terms, then, if your body won't let leptin do its job, you're hungry (Figure 2.08).

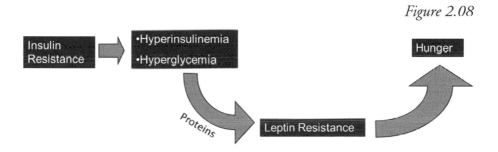

Figure 2.08

If you're confused about why you often eat when you feel full or aren't hungry, it's because your leptin has lost the ability to regulate your appetite. The more you eat, the worse the hyperinsulinemia and hyperglycemia get, and the hungrier you are, so you eat still more, and of course then you gain weight.

Three other metabolic disorders are bound together with leptin resistance and insulin resistance. Because you have a high level of circulating insulin, your sympathetic nervous system is stimulated, causing your kidneys to retain salt in your blood.

Figure 2.09

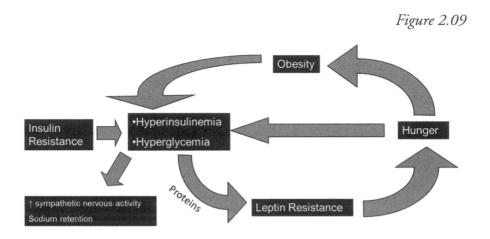

Your volume of circulating blood is about 5 liters. Your blood is in a closed system. When you have the right amount of fluid in your circulatory system, your blood pressure is normal. When your kidneys start retaining salt in your circulating blood, water is drawn into the circulatory system. The salt pulls water into a closed system causing a volume increase, and as the volume increases, blood pressure begins to rise. Thus insulin resistance has caused high blood pressure, or hypertension (Figure 2.10).

Figure 2.10

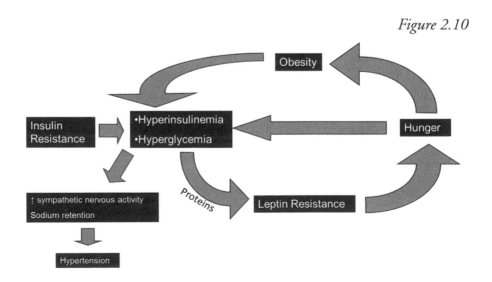

In our studies, insulin resistance was the cause of high blood pressure in 60 percent of people we saw who had hypertension.

It has also been shown that insulin resistance causes high levels of triglycerides (harmful cholesterol) and low levels of HDL (healthy cholesterol). As a result of your insulin resistance, you may have unhealthy cholesterol levels as well as and hypertension. Furthermore, your insulin resistance can progress to the point where it causes you to develop type 2 diabetes.

Figure 2.11

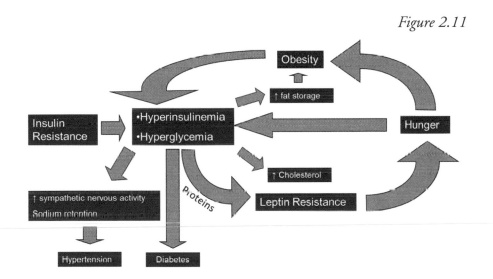

So, how do you correct the insulin resistance that triggers this metabolic disaster? Go for a walk. Walk rapidly enough that you almost break a sweat. If you do this every day for an hour, 7 days per week for 2 weeks, you can break the cycle, eliminate your insulin resistance, and bring your body back into balance. Another way to break the cycle is by going to a gym and breaking a sweat for 1 hour 5 days per week.

So, to sum up: You most likely became insulin resistant because you were overweight and sedentary. If you're overweight and exercise regularly, you probably don't have insulin resistance, but few people who are overweight exercise regularly.

Exercising will break up your insulin resistance. People whose weight is normal can also have insulin resistance if they're sedentary. And there are other conditions that can cause insulin resistance. Women with polycystic ovary syndrome have insulin resistance. Such drugs as beta blockers, diuretics, corticosteroids, glucosamine, and many others can cause insulin resistance. If you must take these drugs, then you must exercise to avoid becoming insulin resistant.

APPENDIX D

STRESS, DEPRESSION, AND CORTISOL

When you have physical stress, emotional stress, or depression, your body undergoes many chemical changes. These changes were designed to help your hunter-gatherer ancestors survive a crisis situation. They're called fight-or-flight responses.

One of those changes happens when the adrenal gland, a small gland on top of the kidney, contracts to cause increased secretion of three substances. Two of these chemicals, norepinephrine and epinephrine, make you more mentally agile and heighten your awareness. The third chemical is cortisol, a corticosteroid.

Many of you have heard of the medications cortisone, prednisone, or prednisolone. All of these medications belong to a class called corticosteroids. Some of you may have even been prescribed these medications to reduce inflammation related to medical conditions. Many patients who take corticosteroids have significant and rapid weight gains. If you suffer from stress, depression, or both, your body produces an excess of these corticosteroids.

As for stress, one can have either acute or chronic stress.

In prehistoric times, when our ancestors who were gathering nuts and berries came across a saber-tooth tiger, they experienced acute stress. Luckily, our ancestors' bodies had this built-in fight-or-flight chemical change that allowed them to think fast and get away. If that ancestor was frightened or, worse, injured, a cortisol burst helped him to function well enough to avoid becoming disabled and tiger food. One way or the other, his acute stress resolved in a relatively short time.

Chronic stress and depression are, however, long-term conditions. They can be caused by physical illness or injury but are more often due to long-standing life and emotional problems. If your problems are financial, work-related, family, or relationship issues, they can be persistent challenges you deal with all day, every day. In response, your body may constantly be producing an overabundance of norepinephrine, epinephrine, and cortisol. As we've pointed out, excess cortisol can make you gain weight, and worse yet, it can cause insulin resistance, moving you into the cycle of high cholesterol, high blood pressure, weight gain, and, eventually, type 2 diabetes (Figure 3.01).

Figure 3.01

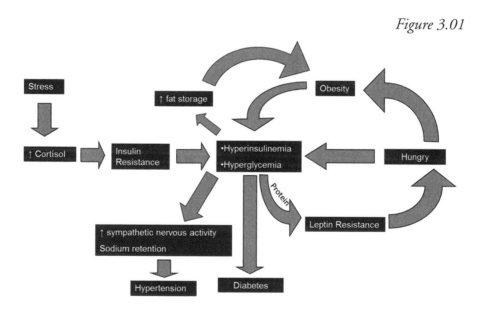

As you can see, the cortisol released in response to stress and depression has triggered a cascade of events. The result is a metabolic disaster, caused by insulin resistance. Fortunately, we know how to break this chain, and it's a fairly simple solution- exercise. Adequate exercise breaks the cycle and allows your body to return to chemical balance.

Remember that you're smarter than you may think. We human beings have an outsized brain for our relatively small bodies. We've been designed to be problem solvers. And, if you apply your problem-solving abilities and get the assistance you need to help you solve a problem, you'll almost always find a solution. That way you eliminate the stress or depression, enabling you to once again function normally.

APPENDIX E

BODY CHEMISTRY AND GRAIN SENSITIVITY

Although there are many nutritional rules that are common to everyone, each of you has different reactions to certain foods. While some of you can tolerate several servings of grains per day, others may not be able to tolerate more than one serving per day. If you notice that your hunger increases on days when you've added grains (even whole grains), you are grain sensitive and must closely monitor your consumption and your reaction to grains. In order to make your nutrition fit your body chemistry, your meal tracking must be accurate and timely. Make sure that, in addition to recording your foods, you also record your feelings of hunger and the times when you feel hungry.

It's normal for you to be hungry at meal time, but if you're hungry 45 minutes after eating a meal or snack containing grains, you'll have to adjust your diet. You can do this in several ways. You can decrease or eliminate your grain consumption, change the timing of your grain consumption, eat more protein with the grains, or only eat the grains with a full meal. Remember, never eat grains as a snack. You'll need to experiment to get it right. Many of our patients were so sensitive to grains they had to remove them completely from their diets.

Signs of grain intolerance are hunger, bloating, heartburn, and fatigue. If you have these symptoms after eating grains or whole grains, your body chemistry does not process grains properly, and you must avoid them.

If you continue to experience hunger at inappropriate times and have tried the solutions mentioned above, you may have to talk to a dietitian familiar with the 20/20 LifeStyles plan, or contact one of our experts. When you make that contact, be sure to have at least a week's meal tracking online for the dietitian to review with you.

In your 20/20 online tracker, or on the 20/20 LifeStyles website under the Resources and Tools tab you can find two very important tools to help you with inappropriate hunger or other issues on the 20/20 LifeStyles plan.

The first is the Weekly Dietitian Review. One of our registered dietitians will review your meal tracker each week, providing comments, feedback, and goals to help you continue to either lose or maintain your weight. This is also a great platform for you to communicate with your dietitian about questions or problems.

The second tool is Ask An Expert. This is a great tool for resolving problems related to hunger or not losing weight. This tool allows you to text a live dietitian or personal trainer with your question. They will respond to you within minutes and answer your questions. You can access these tools at:

www.2020lifestyles.com/get-started/get-started-online/pricing.aspx

APPENDIX F

COOKING VEGETABLES TO PERFECTION

One of the easiest ways to get healthier and slimmer is to eat more colorful vegetables. The more colorful your plate, the more vitamins, minerals, phytochemicals, and antioxidants you will consume with your food. Selecting your vegetables according to the season can help you both increase variety and enjoy fruits and vegetables at their peak freshness and quality. Here's a guide to the best produce to buy for each season.

Summer: Tomatoes, squash, bell peppers, eggplant, leafy greens, melons, berries, peaches, apricots, cherries, and grapes.

Fall: Broccoli, carrots, cauliflower, spinach, pumpkin, sweet potatoes, beets, kale, apples, bananas, oranges, pears, kiwi, grapefruit, and tangerines.

Winter: Snow peas, winter squash (acorn, butternut, pumpkin), radishes, Brussels sprouts, and avocado.

Spring: Asparagus, onions, artichokes, strawberries, cantaloupe, papaya, pineapple.

Bringing Out The Flavor And Health In Your Vegetables

Season vegetables with a pinch—less than $\frac{1}{10}$ teaspoon—of kosher salt and freshly ground black pepper during the cooking process, not at the end (if you have high blood pressure, do not add salt). Use fresh herbs such as thyme, basil, dill, mint, parsley, cilantro, oregano, or tarragon for some salt-free ways to add flavor. Lemon juice and lime

344

juice can brighten the flavors of vegetables, and flavored vinegars are also wonderful ways to add flavor without excess sodium and calories.

Cooking Techniques

Pairing vegetables with the right cooking technique brings out the best flavor and texture of each one. In many cases, it can preserve the maximum nutrient benefit. For example, slow roasting of carrots brings out more flavor and their natural sweetness.

Chopping Vegetables

The best knife for chopping vegetables is a chef's knife, the workhorse of the knife set. Look for knives made of high-carbon stainless steel. The carbon allows the knife to be sharpened, while the stainless steel keeps the knife from rusting.

When a recipe calls for coarsely chopped vegetables, it usually means cut in pieces more than ¼ inch in size. Finely chopped means smaller than ¼ inch, and minced means even smaller. The term "diced" means cut into perfect cubes, which can range in size from to ¼ inch. It's important to cut vegetables into uniform pieces so they cook evenly.

Some vegetables can be prepared without a cutting tool. For example, with fresh asparagus, you can remove the tougher bottom part of each spear by grasping it about the middle with forefinger and thumb of one hand, holding the bottom half firmly with thumb and forefinger of the other hand, and bend the spear until it snaps. The tougher bottom will naturally separate from the tender top.

Boiling Vegetables

Boiling is one of the most common methods of cooking with liquid, usually water. Boiling technically happens at 212° F and requires a large amount of water so that when the food is added, the temperature of the water can be maintained. Blanching is another common technique in cooking vegetables. Hot water is also used for blanching, but with the vegetable left in the hot liquid for a much shorter time to avoid cooking it fully. Blanching green vegetables, then shocking them in ice water, makes them more palatable and maintains their vibrant green color. It's also a great way prevent the loss of such nutrients as B vitamins. Because green vegetables, for example, broccoli, easily lose their green color, it's important to cut them into small enough pieces that they cook within 7 minutes. If you don't plan to serve the green vegetables immediately, it's a good idea to plunge them into an ice-water bath once they're boiled. This will stop the cooking and preserve their green color. Once they're cooled, they can then be dried and refrigerated until needed.

Steaming Vegetables

In steam cooking, the hot vapor from a small amount of boiling water is used to cook vegetables. It's a very healthful way of cooking, because vegetables that aren't submersed in hot water are more likely to retain their vitamins and minerals. The best way to steam vegetables is in a pan with an upper steamer basket, so the food is prevented from touching the water and thereby losing its nutrients. For steaming, vegetables need to be cut in uniform pieces of small to medium size so that they cook quickly and evenly. This is particularly important for cruciferous vegetables such as cauliflower and broccoli, which can give off unpleasant odors if overcooked. Try steaming carrots, green beans, leafy greens, and other tender vegetables. Try adding aromatic spices like cinnamon sticks, lemongrass, and ginger to the steaming liquid to infuse subtle flavors.

Stir-Frying Vegetables

Stir-frying is a great way to cook vegetables quickly while preserving nutrients. Be mindful, however, of the oil used in stir-frying when you calculate portion size. Too much oil in the pan before you cook the vegetables can add unwanted calories to a healthy dish.

Since stir-frying is a quick-cooking technique, it's important to have all the ingredients for the dish prepared and organized before you start cooking. This means that before you begin to cook, you must cut your meats, vegetables, and other ingredients in bite-size pieces in advance, and these pieces must also be dry so they don't steam when placed in the pan. Liquids, such as low-sodium soy sauce, rice wine vinegar, and chicken stock should also be ready at hand. Traditional Chinese stir-frying is done in a wok-a bowl-shaped skillet-but it can also be done in a large sauté pan as long as the bottom is thick enough to distribute the high heat evenly. Whether you're using a wok or sauté pan, get it really hot before you add any of the ingredients. Use an oil with a high smoke point, such as canola oil or peanut oil. Don't use a nonstick pan. These aren't generally meant for use at temperatures above 500°F.

After the pan is heated, add some of your oil, being sure to measure no more than 1 teaspoon per serving. Also be aware that you can stir-fry items in water instead of oil, to reduce the fat and calorie content of the meal.

Many stir-fry recipes begin with the addition of seasonings such as garlic, chili peppers, or ginger and cooking them for a short time, about 10 seconds. Other ingredients, which take longer to cook, are added next. Because home-use woks are smaller, you may need to cook in batches, then finally bring all the ingredients together for a minute or two to allow the flavors to blend. So, for example, you may cook your thin slices of chicken or beef until almost done, remove and set them aside, then cook your string beans, then return the meat with sauce ingredients to bring the entire dish together.

Vegetables that are wonderful to add to a stir- include bell peppers, broccoli, carrots, mushrooms, onions, and sugar snap or snow peas.

Roasting Vegetables

Roasting vegetables such as green beans, asparagus, cauliflower, and broccoli brings out their natural sweetness and gives them an appealing golden color. Begin with uniform cuts of your vegetables and spread on a shallow baking pan in a consistent even layer without crowding. Drizzle a slight amount of extra virgin olive oil and a light sprinkle of kosher salt and pepper. Toss to make sure all the pieces are coated. Roast at 450° F for 15-20 minutes, or until golden brown. Sprinkle lightly with parmesan cheese for added flavor. Try roasting carrots, to bring out the natural sugars, and add a dash of cinnamon for a sweet, yet healthy, side dish.

Grilling Vegetables

Just like roasting, grilling your vegetables locks in flavor and caramelizes them to give them a crispy sweetness. Grilling is delicious way to prepare corn, sweet potatoes, zucchini, squash, onions, and asparagus. A good way to tell whether your grill is hot enough for cooking is to hold your hand about 6 inches above the cooking surface. If you can hold it there for more than 6 seconds, you have a low fire; 5 seconds a medium fire; less than 3 seconds a hot fire. While the grill is heating up, clean the grate with a stiff wire brush, then spray it with vegetable oil spray to prevent the food from sticking. Although most vegetables don't need precooking before going on the grill, some denser ones, such as artichokes and eggplant, do. Holding the vegetable pieces with tongs, place them directly on the grill or in a grilling basket. Allow them to be heated evenly by turning and rotating them over the hot grill. Once they're tender and golden, remove them from the heat. Try grilling asparagus, bell peppers, and mushrooms to add variety to your meals.

Sautéing Vegetables

If you sauté vegetables, you'll be cooking quickly and easily with relatively little oil. You can also easily sauté in water to avoid extra calories. This is a great way to retain the food's vitamins, minerals, flavor, and color. Ideal vegetables to sauté include tender ones such as asparagus, baby artichokes, snow peas, sweet peppers, onions, and mushrooms. Cut your vegetables into bite-size pieces so they and cook evenly and quickly. Heat your sauté pan over high heat, add the oil, and in a few seconds when the oil begins to shimmer, add your vegetables. Toss them over the heat and cook them until they are tender. Cooking time will depend on the desired tenderness and characteristics of the vegetables.

APPENDIX G

THE IMPORTANCE OF WATER IN YOUR PLAN

It's important that you drink 2 quarts (64 ounces) of water per day. Water is your most important nutrient. You could live without food for weeks, but if you're without water for a few days, you'll die. Almost all the major systems in your body need water to function. How does water help your body? It does the following things:

-Regulates body temperature

-Keeps tissue in the eyes, mouth, and nose moist and healthy

-Lubricates joints

-Keeps body organs healthy

-Helps eliminate metabolic waste products and bowel endotoxins

-Allows the kidneys to function

-Helps transport minerals and nutrients to tissue

-Carries oxygen to the cells

-Keeps blood volume at an adequate level for life

-Keeps blood viscosity low enough to be circulated

-Helps prevent infection

-Help maintain the "good" bacteria in your intestines

-Keeps fluid level in the brain, spine, etc., so it can act as a shock absorber

So, as you can see, keeping adequately hydrated is vital for health. But because the body has a very limited ability to store water, it must have its water stores replenished daily.

The 20/20 LifeStyles plan puts additional demands on your hydration. In the first few weeks of the plan, most of you will lose weight quite rapidly. Initially, when you reduce your caloric intake, your body burns your stored glycogen (a type of stored carbohydrate). Glycogen has an affinity for water, and when you burn the glycogen, the water is released. This could cause your body to become dehydrated.

Dehydration causes a drop in your metabolic rate

Even a 1 percent reduction in adequate hydration can bring about a reduction in muscle function. And because muscles are your prime means of burning calories, any reduction in their performance will slow your metabolism and your weight loss.

Burning fat creates waste products, and these wastes, including ammonia, urea, and uric acid, can be toxic to your body. They are, however, water soluble, and drinking adequate water helps eliminate them from your body.

Protein metabolism also produces ketones as a waste product. Drinking adequate water helps flush these ketones out of your system and keeps your organs healthy.

We've mentioned that water is necessary to maintain blood volume. Now, blood carries oxygen and nutrients to your muscles, and if your muscles have an inadequate blood supply, they'll be less efficient and will burn fewer calories. Dehydration can also cause muscle damage, if the muscles should go into spasm.

The 20/20 LifeStyles plan is relatively high in fiber. High-fiber diets are healthy for a number of reasons, but without adequate hydration, they can lead to constipation.

We frequently misinterpret thirst for hunger. Keeping hydrated eliminates that hunger. Additionally, drinking water during a meal helps you feel full sooner.

Since you will be exercising 5 or more times a week, you will be losing a great deal of water in perspiration. This water needs to be replaced.

In warmer climates or in summer months you lose more water through evaporation, so it is even more important to keep up your water consumption at those times.

Some fruits and vegetables have fairly high water contents, as do some other foods. These help with keeping you hydrated. On the other hand, coffee, tea, caffeinated drinks, and alcohol are diuretics and actually cause you to be more dehydrated.

The easiest way to get plenty of water is to drink 8 ounces of water 8 times per day. That will keep you well hydrated and help your weight loss.

To make it easier to consume enough water, try some of the following:

- **Drink good-tasting water:** Water in various locations varies in quality. Find a water that tastes good to you. In some locations tap water is adequate, but in others you may need to use a water-filtration system or bottled water to make your water taste great.

- **Carry a container with you:** Choose a container that is convenient and attractive. Have it with you all day, and train yourself to use it.

- **Track your water:** Use your meal tracker to record your water consumption.

- **Flavor your water:** Use lemons, limes, or cucumbers to add pleasant flavor to your water.

- **Treat yourself with water:** When dining out, try carbonated mineral water with a twist of lemon or lime, instead of an alcoholic drink. Sample different brands, and see which you like the best.

- **Caffeine dehydrates you:** Soda drinks, tea, and coffee with caffeine actually take water from your body. THEY ARE NOT SUBSTITUTES FOR WATER.

Give water a fresh look, because it really does do the body good!

APPENDIX H

TASTY RECIPES FOR EACH STAGE OF THE 20/20 LIFESTYLES PLAN

Here are some tasty recipes to help get you started experimenting with healthy foods. We've organized them by the stages of the plan, so they fit perfectly with your meal plan at each stage. Videos with more recipes and cooking tips for each stage can be found in Appendix J.

STAGE 1 RECIPES

Avocado Tuna Salad

This protein-based entrée is a great way to include healthy fat with your very lean protein. This recipe is quick, easy, and makes a great no-heat lunch.

Ingredients:

- ☐ 1 12 ounce can chunk light tuna in water, drained and flaked
- ☐ ⅛ avocado
- ☐ ¼ cup reduced-fat mayo
- ☐ 3 teaspoons lemon juice
- ☐ 1½ teaspoons chopped oregano

Directions:

Combine ingredients in a medium bowl and mix until blended well.

Serves 3. Per serving: calories 173, fat 6.5 g, carbohydrate 5 g, protein 26.5 g.

* Remember to limit tuna consumption to 2 servings per week.

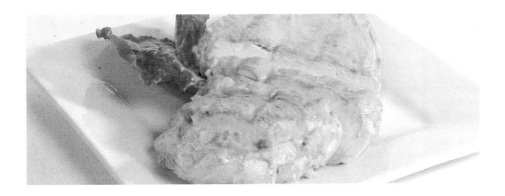

Baked Poupon Chicken

This dish, definitely a crowd favorite, proves that lean protein can be flavorful. Use this as a main entrée for Stage 1, and for Stage 2, add a side of fresh vegetables for a complete meal.

Ingredients:

- ☐ 4 tablespoons Grey Poupon Dijon mustard
- ☐ 1½ tablespoons olive oil
- ☐ 1-2 cloves minced garlic
- ☐ ½ teaspoon Italian seasoning
- ☐ 1 ⅓ pound boneless skinless chicken breasts

Directions:

- Preheat oven to 375° F.

- Mix mustard, oil, garlic, and seasoning in a large bowl. Add chicken and mix to coat.

- Place chicken in baking pan. Bake 20 minutes, or until chicken meat turns white.

Serves 4. Per serving: calories 230, fat 8 g, carbohydrate 2 g, protein 36 g.

STAGE 2 RECIPES

Spaghetti Squash

Spaghetti squash is an outstanding pasta substitute. Use it in a traditional spaghetti dish, stir fry, or just add a healthy fat serving and use it as a side dish.

Basic cooking instructions (oven or microwave):

Oven: Pierce the whole shell several times with a large fork or skewer and place in baking dish. Cook squash in a preheated 375° F (190° C) oven for approximately 1 hour or until flesh is tender.

Microwave: Cut the squash in half, lengthwise. Remove the seeds and place the squash with open side down in a microwave dish using ¼ cup of water. Cover with plastic wrap and cook on high for 10-12 minutes.

Once cooked, halve the squash and use a fork to scrape out its fibrous flesh into spaghetti-like strands.

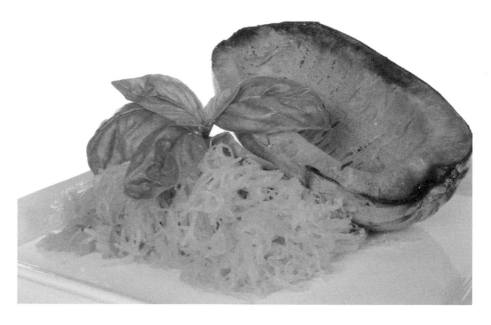

Spaghetti Squash Marinara

This recipe is a great low-calorie pasta alternative. Add your favorite vegetables or lean protein to make it a complete meal. Makes 4 servings.

Ingredients:

- ☐ 1 small spaghetti squash (about 2 pounds)
- ☐ 1 28 ounce can no-salt-added diced tomatoes
- ☐ 1 tablespoon extra virgin olive oil
- ☐ ½ cup finely chopped onion
- ☐ 2 cloves garlic, finely chopped
- ☐ 1 pinch dried red pepper flakes
- ☐ ½ teaspoon salt
- ☐ ½ teaspoon dried basil
- ☐ ⅓ teaspoon dried oregano
- ☐ dash freshly ground black pepper

Directions:

- Cook spaghetti squash using either the oven or microwave method as above.

- Heat oil in a medium skillet over medium-high heat. Add onion and sauté until translucent, about 4 minutes. Mix in the garlic and cook another 2 minutes, stirring constantly. Add tomatoes, red pepper flakes, salt, basil, and oregano. Cook, stirring until the tomatoes are tender and floating in juices but still hold their shape, about 5 minutes. Season with black pepper.

- Halve the baked squash horizontally. Scrape out and discard the seeds. Using a fork, scrape out the squash in strands.

- Divide 4 cups of squash among 4 deep pasta bowls. Spoon ¼ of the sauce over the squash in each bowl.

- Top with very lean or lean protein, or sauté vegetables with ground turkey breast to add protein.

Serves 4. Per serving: calories 150, fat 5 g, carbohydrate 28 g, protein 3 g.

Recipe from Calorieking.com

Coconut Lime Cauliflower "Rice"

Using cauliflower as a substitute for rice is a wonderful way to add fiber and volume to a dish without adding excess calories or carbohydrates. Use this dish along with grilled tilapia or salmon.

Ingredients:

- ☐ 1 large head cauliflower (stems and leaves removed), separated into pieces
- ☐ ½ cup fresh cilantro, chopped
- ☐ Juice of ½ lime
- ☐ 1 tablespoon olive oil
- ☐ 1 tablespoon minced garlic
- ☐ 2 tablespoons light coconut milk, canned
- ☐ ⅛ teaspoon salt

Directions:

Rinse cauliflower and dry well with paper towels. Next, "rice" your cauliflower by either pulsing it in a food processor, taking care not to overprocess into a purée, or grating it with a fine cheese grater. Heat oil in a large sauce pan over medium heat, then add in cauliflower "rice," chopped cilantro, lime juice, and garlic. Cook until cauliflower is hot throughout, then add coconut milk and a pinch of salt. Cook for an additional 2 minutes, then serve warm.

Serves 4. Per serving: calories 74, fat 3 g, carbohydrates 8.5 g, protein 3 g, sodium 117 mg.

Roasted Cauliflower With Rosemary And Garlic

This side dish is a perfect companion to a piece of grilled salmon or chicken. Roasting vegetables is a great way to bring out flavor without adding extra calories.

Ingredients:

- ☐ 1 large head cauliflower (stems and leaves removed), cut into florets
- ☐ 3 tablespoons water
- ☐ 1 tablespoon olive oil
- ☐ 3 cloves garlic, crushed
- ☐ 1 teaspoon dried rosemary, or 1 tablespoon fresh rosemary
- ☐ ½ teaspoon kosher salt (optional)

Directions:

- Preheat oven to 450° F.

- Toss together all the ingredients in shallow casserole or rimmed baking sheet.

- Place in center of oven and bake for 15 minutes. Stir and continue to bake about 15 minutes longer until the cauliflower is tender and brown in spots.

Serves 6. Per serving: calories 50, fat 2.5 g, carbohydrate 6 g, protein 3 g.

Recipe from 1,000 Low fat Recipes by Terry Blonder Golson

STAGE 3 RECIPES

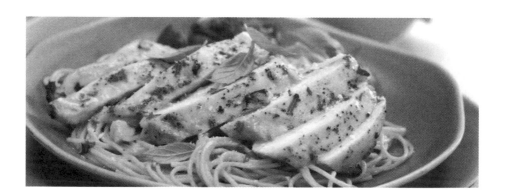

Chicken And Vegetable Pasta

This recipe is another of our favorites. Shirataki noodles, made from tofu, are a low-calorie and tasty substitute for pasta.

Ingredients:

- ☐ 2 8 ounce bags shirataki tofu noodles
- ☐ 8 ounces raw boneless, skinless, lean chicken breast cutlets
- ☐ ⅛ teaspoon oregano
- ☐ ⅛ teaspoon thyme
- ☐ ¼ teaspoon salt, divided (34)
- ☐ ¼ teaspoon black pepper
- ☐ 20 asparagus spears, cut into 1 inch pieces (about 2½ cups)
- ☐ 1 cup sliced mushrooms
- ☐ ¼ cup sun-dried tomatoes, thinly sliced
- ☐ 2 teaspoons chopped garlic
- ☐ 1 tablespoon light whipped butter or light buttery spread
- ☐ 1 tablespoon Parmesan-style grated topping

34. "Divided means spread evenly, not just "dumped" in.

Directions:

- Use a strainer to rinse and drain noodles well. Pat dry. Cut noodles into smaller pieces and set aside.

- Spray skillet with nonstick spray and bring to medium-high heat on the stovetop. Add chicken and season with oregano, thyme, $1/8$ teaspoon salt, and pepper. Cook for about 4 minutes per side until fully cooked (no pink).

- Remove chicken from skillet. When cool enough to handle, slice chicken into strips and set aside.

- Remove skillet from heat, respray, and return to medium-high heat. Add asparagus and 2 tablespoons water. Cover and cook for 4 minutes.

- Remove cover and add mushrooms, tomatoes, and garlic to the skillet. Stirring occasionally, cook until vegetables are tender, about 4 minutes.

- Add noodles to skillet, stir, and cook just until excess water has evaporated and noodles are hot, about 2 minutes.

- Add butter, remaining $1/8$ teaspoon salt, and sliced chicken to the skillet. Cook and stir until ingredients are well mixed and butter has melted, about 1 minute.

- Add parmesan and mix well.

Serves 2. Per serving: 274 calories, fat 8 g, sodium 546 mg, carbohydrates 19 g, fiber 8 g, protein 34 g.

Adapted from Hungry-Girl.com recipe

Crustless Smoked Salmon Quiche With Dill

This dish is a great way to incorporate protein into a baked dish. Use as a dinner entrée or tasty breakfast.

Ingredients:

- ☐ 1¼ cups fat-free evaporated milk
- ☐ ¼ cup fat-free sour cream
- ☐ 1 teaspoon Dijon mustard
- ☐ 4 large egg whites
- ☐ 1 large egg
- ☐ ½ cup (2 ounces) shredded Cabot 50 percent Light cheese
- ☐ ½ cup thinly sliced green onions
- ☐ ¼ cup smoked salmon, chopped (about 2 ounces)
- ☐ 2 tablespoons chopped fresh dill
- ☐ ½ teaspoon black pepper
- ☐ Cooking spray

Directions:

- Preheat oven to 350°. Combine first 5 ingredients in a large bowl and whisk. Stir in cheese, onions, salmon, dill, and pepper. Pour egg mixture into 9 inch pie plate coated with cooking spray. Bake at 350° for 35 minutes. Let stand 15 minutes.

- Serve this warm from the oven or chilled.

Serves 2. Per serving: calories 340, fat 9 g, carbohydrate 28 g, protein 36 g.

STAGE 4 RECIPES

Cauliflower Crust Hawaiian Pizza

This recipe features a new take on pizza, using cauliflower as a great low-calorie pizza crust. Use the crust recipe and customize the toppings however you would like. Adding 4 ounces of chicken strips to make a BBQ chicken pizza is another great variation of this recipe.

Ingredients:

Crust:

- ☐ ½ large head cauliflower, shredded, makes approximately 2 cups
- ☐ 1 large egg
- ☐ 1 cup finely shredded part-skim mozzarella cheese
- ☐ 1 teaspoon dried oregano
- ☐ ½ teaspoon dried minced garlic
- ☐ ½ teaspoon onion salt

Toppings: (can adjust per taste, though nutritionals listed below will change)

- ☐ ½ cup tomato-basil marinara sauce
- ☐ ½ cup finely shredded part-skim mozzarella cheese
- ☐ 3 slices Canadian bacon, cut into strips
- ☐ ½ cup pineapple tidbits

Directions:

- Shred cauliflower into small crumbles. If you use a food processor, make sure you stop at crumbles, not purée. You'll need a total of 2 cups or so. Place cauliflower crumbles in large bowl and microwave them (dry) for 8 minutes. Let cauliflower cool.

363

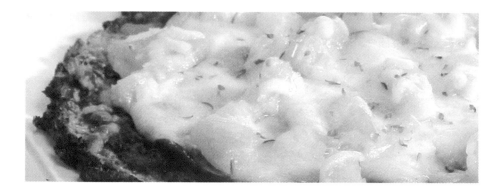

- Preheat oven to 450° F. Spray cookie sheet or pizza pan with nonstick spray (or use a nonstick surface). In medium bowl, mix cauliflower crumbles (now about 1½ cups, as they shrink after cooking) with remaining crust ingredients. Pat the crust into a 9- to 12 inch round on prepared pan. Spray crust lightly with nonstick spray and bake for 15 minutes, or until golden. Remove crust from the oven and turn the heat up to Broil.

- Spread the sauce on top of baked crust, leaving a ½ inch border around the edge. Sprinkle ¼ cup cheese on top. Add bacon and pineapple, spreading it out around the pizza. Sprinkle remaining cheese on top. Broil pizza 3-4 minutes or until toppings are hot and cheese is melted and bubbly. Cut into 6 slices and serve immediately.

Serves 6. Per serving: calories 151, fat 7 g, saturated fat 4 g, protein 13 g, carbohydrates 9 g, fiber 2 g.

Adapted from recipegirl.com

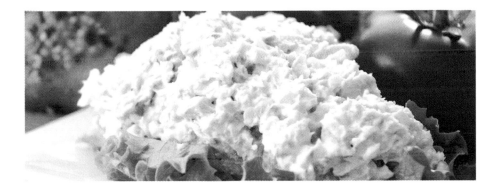

Light Chicken Salad

This dish is great for use as a lean protein source including a healthy fat serving. Serve with whole-wheat wraps, pitas, or atop a large salad for a grain-free option. Classic chicken salads are a great quick meal or lunch. This recipe is a healthier version.

Ingredients:

- ☐ 10 ounces chopped precooked chicken (for vegetarian option, use same portion of Beyond Meat)
- ☐ ⅓ cup red seedless grapes, halved
- ☐ ½ cup diced celery
- ☐ ¼ cup slivered or sliced almonds, toasted
- ☐ ¼ cup 0 percent plain Greek yogurt
- ☐ ¼ cup low-fat mayo
- ☐ 1 teaspoon fresh squeezed lemon juice
- ☐ 2 tablespoons minced chives
- ☐ Dash black pepper

Directions: Mix all ingredients in a bowl.

Serves 2. Per serving: Calories 287, fat 7.5 g, sat fat 0.5 g, carbohydrates 12 g, protein 36.5 g, fiber 3 g, sodium about 123 mg.

STAGE 5 RECIPES

Curried Chicken Breasts

This recipe features a flavorful way to include yogurt in cooking. Note, advance prep is required, as chicken must marinate at least 30 minutes before baking.

Ingredients:

- ☐ 2 pounds boneless, skinless chicken breasts
- ☐ ½ cup plain nonfat yogurt
- ☐ 3 tablespoons lemon juice
- ☐ 1 tablespoon low-sodium soy sauce
- ☐ 2 teaspoons curry powder

Directions:

- Preheat oven to 375° F.

- Combine yogurt, lemon juice, soy sauce, and curry. Pour over chicken and let sit at room temperature 30 minutes, or in refrigerator for several hours.

- Bake for 40 minutes or until chicken meat turns white.

Serves 6. calories 180, fat 2 g, carbohydrate 3 g, protein 36 g.

Recipe adapted from Low on the Go by Terri Petersen

Tandoori Chicken

A delicious version of a classic dish, and another great way to use yogurt for cooking. Serve alongside your favorite steamed vegetable. Note, advance prep is required. Chicken must marinate for at least 6 hours.

Ingredients:

- ☐ 1 cup plain nonfat yogurt
- ☐ 1 tablespoon finely minced or grated gingerroot
- ☐ 2 large cloves garlic, peeled and minced
- ☐ 1 tablespoon paprika (use some hot paprika, if desired)
- ☐ 1½ teaspoons coriander
- ☐ 1½ teaspoons cumin
- ☐ 1 teaspoon freshly ground black pepper
- ☐ ¾ teaspoon cayenne, or to taste
- ☐ 2 pounds boneless skinless chicken breast

Directions:

- In a small bowl, combine marinade ingredients.

- Make interval slashes 1 inch deep in chicken. Coat chicken pieces with marinade, rubbing some marinade into the slashes. Place the chicken in a bowl, cover bowl tightly with plastic wrap, and refrigerate to marinate for at least 6 hours or up to 24 hours.

- Oil the broiler rack and place it 6 inches from the heat. Preheat the broiler.

- Place chicken pieces on rack and broil for 20 minutes on one side. Turn the pieces over and broil them on the other side for 15 minutes, or until their juices run clear when pierced with a fork.

Serves 6 (approximately 5-oz portions). Per serving: Calories 200, fat 2.5 g, carbohydrate 5 g, protein 38 g.

Recipe adapted from Jane Brody's Good Food Gourmet

STAGE 6 RECIPES

Red Pepper Hummus

Pair this tasty dish with some fresh vegetables, or use it as a sandwich spread.

Ingredients:

- ☐ 1 red bell pepper
- ☐ 2½ tablespoons fresh lemon juice
- ☐ 1 tablespoon tahini (sesame seed paste)
- ☐ ¼ teaspoon freshly ground black pepper
- ☐ ½ teaspoon salt
- ☐ ¼ teaspoon ground cumin
- ☐ 1 15 ounce can garbanzo beans, rinsed and drained
- ☐ 1 garlic clove, minced

Directions:

- Preheat broiler. Halve bell pepper lengthwise and discard seeds and membranes. Place pepper halves, skin side up, on foil-lined baking sheet and flatten with hand. Broil 10 minutes or until blackened. Place in a zip-top plastic bag and seal. Let stand 10 minutes, then peel skins. Combine bell pepper with remaining ingredients in food processor and process until smooth.

Serves 8 (¼ cup servings). Per serving: Calories 60, fat 2 g, carbohydrate 9 g, protein 3 g.

Slow-Cooker White Chili

This flavorful version of a classic dish featuring chicken and white beans is a perfect way to combine protein and carbohydrates. To add a healthy fat, top with ⅛ avocado.

Ingredients:

- ☐ 2 15 ounce cans Great Northern beans, drained
- ☐ 20 ounces cooked, shredded chicken breasts
- ☐ 1 cup onions
- ☐ 1½ cups chopped yellow, red, or green bell pepper
- ☐ 2 garlic cloves, minced
- ☐ 2 teaspoons cumin
- ☐ ½ teaspoon salt
- ☐ ½ teaspoon dried oregano
- ☐ 3½ cups nonfat chicken broth (2 14-oz cans)
- ☐ Cayenne pepper
- ☐ 1 tablespoon light sour cream
- ☐ ¼ cup reduced-fat mozzarella cheese

Directions:

- Combine all ingredients except cayenne pepper, sour cream, and cheese in slow cooker and cover. Cook on low for 8-10 hours, or on high for 4-5 hours.
- Add cayenne pepper and stir. Ladle into bowls and top individual servings with ¼ cup shredded mozzarella and 1 tablespoon light sour cream.

Serves 6. Per serving: Calories 280, fat 4.5 g, carbohydrate 25 g, protein 39 g.

Hummus

Hummus makes a great snack when paired with crisp vegetables such as celery, carrots, jicama, broccoli, or whole-grain crackers. It can also be used as a sandwich spread.

Ingredients:

- ☐ 1 15 ounce can garbanzo beans (chickpeas)
- ☐ ¼ cup tahini (sesame paste)
- ☐ ¼ cup lemon juice
- ☐ Water, if needed
- ☐ 3 large cloves garlic, peeled and crushed
- ☐ ½ teaspoon ground coriander
- ☐ ¼ teaspoon cumin
- ☐ ¼ teaspoon paprika
- ☐ Dash cayenne pepper
- ☐ ¼ cup minced scallions
- ☐ 2 tablespoons minced fresh parsley for garnish

Directions:

- In a blender, in batches, or in a food processor, process chickpeas, tahini, and lemon juice until mixture reaches consistency of a coarse paste. Use as much of the chickpea liquid and/or water as needed.

- Add garlic, coriander, cumin, paprika, and cayenne and process again to combine ingredients thoroughly. Transfer hummus to a bowl and stir in scallions.

- Cover the hummus and chill until 1 hour before serving, adding parsley garnish at last minute.

Serves 14 (2 tablespoon servings). Per serving: Calories 50; fat 3 g; carbohydrate 6 g; protein 2 g.

Recipe adapted from Jane Brody's Good Food Gourmet

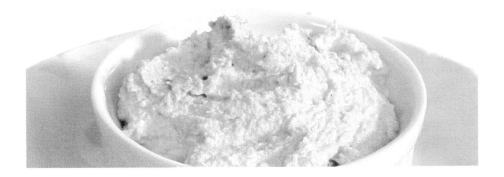

Spicy Edamame Dip

This dip makes a great appetizer to pair with a vegetable tray or shrimp.

Ingredients:

- ☐ 4 large garlic cloves
- ☐ 1 bag (16 ounces) edamame beans
- ☐ 1¼ teaspoons salt (optional)
- ☐ ½ teaspoon ground coriander
- ☐ ½ teaspoon ground cayenne
- ☐ ¼ teaspoon ground cumin
- ☐ ¼ cup olive oil
- ☐ ¼ cup fresh lime juice
- ☐ ¼ cup chopped fresh cilantro, plus a few sprigs for garnish

Directions:

- Roast garlic in an ungreased skillet over medium heat, turning frequently until soft (dark splotches in spots), about 15 minutes. Cool and slip off the paperlike skins.

- Boil edamame beans in salted water to cover until tender, about 5 minutes. Reserve about 1 cup of the cooking water. Drain edamame and cool to room temperature.

- Drop peeled garlic into blender or food processor with the motor running to chop it coarsely. Add drained edamame, salt, and spices. Process, adding ½-¾ cup of cooking water for smooth purée. Add oil, lime juice, and cilantro. Pulse to combine.

- Spoon into serving dish and garnish with cilantro sprigs. Serve at room temperature with cut-up vegetables or shrimp.

Serves 10. Per serving: Calories 120; fat 9 g; carbohydrate 6 g; protein 6 g.

Recipe adapted from wholefoodsmarket.com. Original recipe by Rick Bayless, Chef of Frontera Grill/Topolobampo

STAGE 7 RECIPES

Coconut Crusted Cod

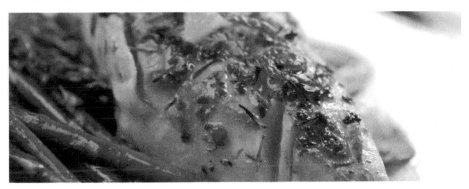

A great way to add extra flavor to white fish without additional calories. Note: tilapia or chicken can be substituted for cod.

Ingredients:

- ☐ 2 slices 100 caloric whole-grain bread, or ⅓ cup whole-grain bread crumbs
- ☐ 4 cod fillets, approximately 5 ounces each, thawed or fresh
- ☐ ⅓ cup unsweetened coconut flakes
- ☐ ¼ teaspoon salt
- ☐ ½ teaspoon garlic powder
- ☐ ¼ teaspoon pepper
- ☐ ⅓ cup liquid egg whites

Directions:

- Preheat oven to 425° F. Line baking pan with foil for easy clean-up and cover with a wire rack, spraying with non-stick oil.

- Cut bread in small pieces and pulse in food processor or blender to fine crumbs, or use 1 /3 cup whole-grain bread crumbs if you have them.

- In a small bowl, combine bread crumbs, salt, garlic, pepper, and shredded coconut and mix. In a separate bowl, whisk egg whites until frothy.

- Dip each cod fillet into egg-white mixture, coating on both sides. Then dip into breadcrumb-coconut mixture, pressing lightly to ensure that both sides are well coated. Place fish on wire rack in baking pan and bake for 17-21 minutes, or until coating is browned and fish is fully cooked.

Serves 4. Per serving: Calories 225, fat 6.5 g, carbohydrates 11 g, protein 31 g, sodium 360 mg.

Recipe adapted from Dashingdish.com.

Asian Turkey Meatballs

A great family-friendly recipe to infuse your protein-centered dish with flavor. Serve alongside stir-fried vegetables or use as a high-protein appetizer.

Ingredients:

- ☐ ¼ cup whole-wheat breadcrumbs
- ☐ 20 ounces ground turkey (99 percent fat-free)
- ☐ 1 egg
- ☐ 1 tablespoon ginger, minced
- ☐ 1 tablespoon garlic, minced
- ☐ ½ tsp salt
- ☐ ¼ cup chopped fresh cilantro
- ☐ 2 green onions, chopped
- ☐ 1 tablespoon low-sodium soy sauce
- ☐ 2 teaspoons sesame oil

Directions:

- Preheat oven to 400° F.

- Combine and mix ground turkey, breadcrumbs, egg, salt, green onions, ginger, garlic, cilantro, soy sauce, and sesame oil, but to retain moistness, don't overmix or compact the mixture.

- Divide mixture into four ¼ cup portions, shape each portion into a ball, and place on baking dish. Bake until cooked through, about 15 minutes.

Serves 4. Per serving: Calories 180, fat 5 g; carbohydrates 4 g, protein 32 g, sodium 550 mg.

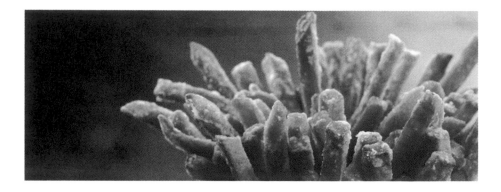

Baked Sweet-Potato "Fries"

Baked sweet potato sticks are a wonderful substitute for a traditional French fry. For a savory variety, add paprika to season. For a sweeter flavor, add cinnamon.

Ingredients:

> 4 medium sweet potatoes, scrubbed
>
> 1 tablespoon extra-virgin olive oil
>
> ¼ teaspoon salt
>
> 2 teaspoons paprika

Directions:

- Preheat oven to 425° F. Slice potatoes in half, then lengthwise to desired thickness for "fries."

- In a medium bowl, mix potatoes with olive oil until evenly coated. Spread potatoes on a baking sheet.

- Sprinkle salt and paprika evenly over potatoes. Bake for about 25 minutes or until soft and cooked through.

Serves 4. Per serving: Calories 131, fat 3.7 g, saturated fat 0.5 g, carbohydrate 23.1 g, protein 1.9 g, sodium 210 mg, fiber 3.6 g, sugar 4.8 g.

Twice-Baked Cheese-and-Broccoli Potatoes

This favorite is a lighter version of a traditional baked potato. Use it as your carbohydrate serving for the meal, alongside your favorite lean protein and nonstarchy vegetable.

Ingredients:

> 4 medium potatoes, scrubbed
>
> 1 cup sharp reduced-fat cheddar cheese
>
> ¼ cup light sour cream
>
> ¼ cup fat-free milk
>
> 4 teaspoons olive oil
>
> 1 teaspoon Dijon mustard
>
> ½ teaspoon salt
>
> ¼ teaspoon cayenne
>
> 3 cups chopped and steamed broccoli florets

Directions:

- Preheat oven to 425° F. Pierce potatoes and bake until skin cracks slightly, about 1 hour. Reduce oven temperature to 375° F.

- Halve potatoes lengthwise. Scoop out pulp, leaving a hollow shell about ¼ inch thick. In a medium bowl, combine pulp with cheese, sour cream, milk, oil, mustard, salt, and cayenne. Fold in broccoli. Spoon mixture into potato shells, place on a baking sheet, and bake until hot and bubbling (about 10 minutes).

Serves 8 (1 serving = 1 loaded potato half). Per serving: Calories 175, fat 5.1 g, saturated fat 1.7 g, carbohydrate 24.8 g, protein 8.6 g, sodium 433 mg, fiber 3.6 g, sugar 2.3 g.

Adapted from Weight Watchers Complete Cookbook

APPENDIX I

SPECIAL CONSIDERATIONS DURING PREGNANCY

If you're pregnant, do not attempt to follow a weight-loss plan. Weight loss during pregnancy is never recommended, so wait until childbirth to begin a meal plan. Even if you're overweight, weight loss during pregnancy is not advisable. You must wait until you are no longer pregnant to begin focusing on weight loss.

Consult your doctor before starting any kind of diet or exercise plan. If you're breastfeeding, your daily calorie needs will be increased. With those increased calorie needs, the easiest way to follow a breastfeeding meal plan is to follow the male meal plans in this book and consume more than 1,500 calories daily. During breastfeeding, rapid weight-loss programs should be avoided, along with severe calorie restriction, to avoid any release into your milk of toxins stored in your body. If you are breastfeeding, consult your doctor before beginning this plan, and keep your total calorie intake above 1,500 calories per day [35].

ALWAYS discuss any exercise plan during pregnancy with your doctor!

Women can and do exercise during pregnancy. What you are capable of during pregnancy depends on the level of your pre-pregnancy exercise and activity, as explained in Chapter 9. Again, always check with your doctor before starting any exercise routine during or just after pregnancy. With your doctor's approval, you may use the following exercise routines:

35. Jan Riordan and Karen Wambach, *Breastfeeding and Human Lactation*, 3rd edition, p. 440

- If you're Level 1 fitness, you can follow the recommended exercise levels for Stages 1-7 during the first six months. For last three months, be sure to discuss the specifics of your exercise plan with your doctor.

- If you're Level 2 fitness, you can follow the recommended exercise levels for Stages 1-6 for the first six months. For the last three months, be sure to discuss the specifics of your exercise plan with your doctor.

- If you're Level 3 fitness, you can follow the recommended exercise levels for Stages 1-3 for the first six months. For the last three months, be sure to discuss the specifics of your exercise plan with your doctor.

Lifestyle plans in pregnancy present some unique issues. If this is your first child, you have no idea of the degree that having a baby will alter your daily life. If this is not your first, the same is still true. Often prospective parents believe they know what it will be like, because they have friends and relatives who have children or have previously had children themselves. But parents in our program have told us repeatedly that even though they thought they were prepared, they were not.

During and after pregnancy, women experience many changes in their body and body chemistry. These changes are very stressful, and the combination of stress, hormonal changes, and altered sleep patterns can be very hard to manage. Usually these stresses subside about 90 days after the pregnancy ends, and good nutrition and exercise can help to minimize the discomfort.

One of the difficult aspects of having a new baby is controlling your time and your daily activities. We've repeatedly discussed time-management issues in this book and how important time management is for controlling your weight and health.

We've found that advance planning and support can make the difference between being in control of your life and feeling overwhelmed. Before the baby's arrival, you must have discussions with your support people (spouse, partner, weight-loss support person, parents, siblings, and children). You should tell them frankly what you will need from them and get their assurances about the level of support they will provide. This is one of many instances where communication is vital to your health and happiness.

If after following these suggestions you're still confused or distressed, talk to your physician or see a psychologist or counselor in your area. If you live in the Puget Sound area, schedule an appointment with one of our psychologists or counselors by calling (425) 462-2776 or by contacting us at: www.proclub.com/Wellness/Counseling

Follow these suggestions for a happy welcoming of your new family member and a rapid recovery from your birthing experience.

APPENDIX J

VIDEOS AVAILABLE FOR ONLINE VIEWING

One of the most important reasons for the success of the 20/20 LifeStyles program is its emphasis on education. As we have repeatedly stated, you've been bombarded with bad information on some topics and find it almost impossible to get any information on other topics. The first step in moving toward long-term success is to educate yourself about your body, your condition, and your nutrition. We recommend viewing several of our videos per week, starting with the free Intro videos. If you live in the Puget Sound area, you should attend the free Introductory Seminar. You'll receive a tremendous amount of information. Call (425) 861-6258 for a reservation or go online at:

www.2020lifestyles.com/get-started.aspx

Share these videos with your family or support group. It will help them understand your weight problem and your solution to that problem. Watching a video is a great way to motivate yourself when you start feeling as if you'd like to go off plan, or when you've had a bad day.

There are more than 60 videos in this series, providing answers, explanations, and motivation online at: www.2020lifestyles.com/resources-tools/educational-videos.aspx

These videos, an excellent means of support, are tailored specifically to the 20/20 LifeStyles plan. Check back periodically as new and revised titles are continuously added. Titles and brief descriptions are listed below.

Free Videos:

- Intro **Seminar 1** (Free)

    Weight gain is not your fault. Meet Dr. Mark Dedomenico and learn the key contributors to weight gain.

- Intro Seminar 2 (Free)

    Learn more about the reasons for weight gain including the hormone ghrelin which sends you searching for food.

- Intro **Seminar 3** (Free)

    Find out about the hormone leptin, a long-term regulator of food intake and how being insulin resistant can lead to weight gain.

- Intro **Seminar 4** (Free)

    Discover how insulin resistance affects the body, what your set point is, and how NEAT is an important part of weight loss.

- Intro Seminar 5 (Free)

  Did you know sugar causes the release of a chemical to your brain's reward center? Learn about Reward Center eating and how to create a healthier lifestyle.

- Intro Seminar 6 (Free)

  Get started with the 20/20 LifeStyles program and our uniquely successful approach to permanent weight loss.

- Stage 1: Protein (Free)

  The focus of this video is on healthy proteins, appropriate serving sizes, and how to easily prepare meal-replacement shakes. Also, learn the first steps in starting an effective exercise program.

- Stage 2: Veggies (Free)

  Integrate vegetables into your diet and discover five simple warm-up activities to enhance your exercise routine.

- Overview of Your Program (Free)

  Learn about the 20/20 meal-plan approach and how each of the weekly stages translates to specific food groups. Find out more about the 20/20 LifeStyles support team including dietitians, trainers, and lifestyle counselors.

Videos for purchase:

Cooking:

- Thinking Outside the Blender- **Stage 1**

  Learn how to make high-protein muffins and pancakes as a nutritional equivalent to drinking your protein shakes.

- Getting Creative with Veggies- Stage 2

  Make delicious recipes loaded with vegetables including broccoli and cherry tomato salad, as well as how to prepare spaghetti squash.

- Adding Choices with Cheese- **Stage 3**

   Discover ways to incorporate cheese or high-protein yogurt into your meal plan. Also, learn how to prepare a crustless smoked salmon quiche with dill.

- Staying Fit with Fruit and Dairy- **Stage 4 &** Stage 5

   Enjoy fruit and dairy in your meal plan through two fabulous meals: salmon with dill sauce and an Asian asparagus and orange salad.

- Boost Your Options with Beans- Stage 6

   Incorporate beans into your diet through tasty recipes including homemade hummus and crab salad with white beans and gourmet greens.

- Whole Grains as a Complement- Stage 7

   Add some variety into your diet by adding back bread and cooked grains. Find out how to make healthy personal pizzas and a Greek quinoa salad.

Exercise:

Exercising and Having Fun

   a. Do you dread the word exercise? You'll learn how to create an exercise plan that is fun and understand the health benefits of being active.

Getting Started:

Stage 3: Cheese

   Get the facts on cheese and learn about the importance of meal tracking. Also, find out how sleep can impact your appetite and weight, and how strength training will benefit your exercise routine.

Stage 4: Fruit

Find out which fruits to avoid, get motivational tips from one of our lifestyle counselors, and learn proper stretching techniques.

Stage 5: Milk and Yogurt

Low fat vs. nonfat-the pros and cons, plus a list of recommended snacks and more tips from one of our lifestyle counselors.

Stage 6: Legumes

Get the scoop on beans along with tasty recipe ideas. Also, keep your muscles loose by learning the secrets of the foam roller.

Stage 7: Whole Grains

Reintroduce whole grains into your diet and get meal and snack ideas. Tips on exercise while traveling and effective goal setting. Spice up your exercise routine with intervals and learn about the concept of reward-center eating.

Lifestyle Series:

- Coping with Celebration

Do you find yourself falling off plan during holidays and celebrations? Learn useful tips and tricks to help you maintain your new healthy lifestyle.

- Grocery Shopping 1

Rediscover the produce section and receive a variety of smart shopping tips.

- Grocery Shopping 2

Find out why healthy protein sources are an indispensable part of your weight-loss plan.

- Grocery Shopping 3

  Get the scoop on which healthy fats and grains to pick up at the grocery store.

- Grocery Shopping 4

  Learn how to decipher food labels. Find out what's hiding in the health food section.

- Creating Healthy Family Lifestyles Habits

  Discover the key factors in developing and maintaining a healthy lifestyle for you and your family. Learn what causes children to be overweight.

- Lapse and Relapse 1

  Learn how to identify and manage situations that lead to a loss of self-control.

- Lapse and Relapse 2

  Learn how controlling your environment can prevent lapses and keep you on track.

- Metabolism and NEAT

  Get the details on Non-Exercise Activity Thermogenesis (NEAT). Find out how NEAT can improve your chances of losing weight.

- Misconceptions About Dieting

  Get the truth about common dieting and exercise myths.

- Planning Around Temptation

  Do you struggle to make healthy choices at fast-food restaurants, parties, and snack time? Learn how planning ahead can help you make better decisions.

- Satiety 1

Discover the recipe of diet, exercise, and lifestyle change that will elevate your energy expenditure and stop your brain from sending hunger signals.

- Satiety 2

Effectively control your metabolism and hunger by consuming certain foods in your diet.

- Self-Monitoring for Success

Meal tracking is the key to successful weight-loss and maintenance. We'll help you to learn how to meal track consistently, managing portion size and overcoming the many obstacles that could get in your way.

- Sleep 1

Sleep-the easiest solution to improving mental performance, weight loss, and overall health.

Sleep 2

A simple change in your diet can affect your sleep patterns and be your solution to improved sleep.

- How To Stay Motivated for Life

Create a visualization plan that keeps you motivated and positive for long-term success.

- Stress 1

Discover how stress directly impacts weight gain.

- Stress 2

Learn about physical, mental, and interpersonal stress responses and how to effectively manage your stressors.

- Stress 3

    Assess the stress in your life, identify warning signals, and create your own stress-related first aid kit.

- Denial

    Overcome your denial and feel better about your health.

- Disordered Eating

    Equip yourself with important information about disordered eating and how these chaotic eating patterns are triggered.

- Dining Right 1

    Learn how to manage the variety of challenges you encounter when eating restaurant meals. Enjoy dining out while dining right!

- Dining Right 2

    Practice mindful eating. Slow down, enjoy your food, and stick with your program.

- Finding Support

    Develop a strong support network to help you maintain a healthy lifestyle and avoid setbacks.

- Fish Oil-The Fountain of Youth

    Discover the benefits of fish oil, including prevention of high blood pressure and many other conditions.

- Vitamins and Minerals 1

    What foods are the good sources of Vitamins C, E, and beta carotene and what are the recommended daily allowances.

- Vitamins and Minerals 2

Discover why you need vitamins and minerals such as folic acid, co-enzyme Q10, calcium, and many more. Are supplements like ginseng and ginkgo biloba really beneficial?

- Water Does a Body Good

How much water does your body need? Learn how water plays an important role in weight loss.

Nutrition:

- Calories Comparison 1

Discover how consuming too much sugar affects your body's chemical balance.

- Calories Comparison 2

Watch out for beverages, appetizers, and side dishes that offer nothing but empty calories.

- Calories Comparison 3

Manage your calorie intake and make good choices even when eating pizza and fast food.

- Carbs and Sugar 1

Learn how consuming refined carbohydrates and sugars will keep you on the constant search for food.

- Carbs and Sugar 2

Don't be tricked by food manufacturers who mislead consumers by referring to sugar by other names in their food products.

- Carbs and Sugar 3

Did you know sweetened beverages disrupt your body's chemical balance and create bad habits?

- Carbs and Sugar 4

  Discover how sugars and other carbs cause you to crave them even more, especially in the afternoon and evening.

- Reward Center 1

  Learn how certain foods stimulate your brain's reward center and how to double your chances of maintaining weight loss.

- Reward Center 2

  Discover how food engineers create foods to arouse your reward center causing you to overeat.

- Reward Center 3

  Why do reward-center foods trigger a cue-craving-reward habit? Learn how to break the cycle.

- Reward Center 4

  Why can't I stop overeating? Learn how to reprogram your brain and replace bad habits with healthy new behaviors.

- Reward Center 5

  Developing if-then cognitive responses is key when encountering and overcoming reward-center foods.

- Reward Center 6

  Practice and perfect your if-then cognitive plans. Discover the acronym HALT NOW.

- Good Fats vs. Bad Fats 1

  Understand the importance of fat in your diet while learning about insulin resistance. Get the scoop on saturated and unsaturated fats.

- Good Fats vs. Bad Fats 2

Get your kitchen in shape to help reduce your fat intake. Learn to prepare healthy low-fat meals with helpful cooking and shopping tips.

APPENDIX K

MEAL-PLAN VARIATIONS FOR ETHNIC DIETS

Any traditional ethnic diet can be adapted and altered to fit the 20/20 LifeStyles food plan. You may adapt your traditional ethnic recipes to fit into your new, healthy lifestyle. If your traditional diet does not include dairy, for example, feel free to omit this from your meal plan. Many ethnic diets revolve around carbohydrates as the main dish, and if that's the case for your diet, you'll need to increase your protein intake and reduce your carbohydrate intake. Your carbohydrate intake needs to be 1 serving per meal, at most. These changes are necessary to develop your new healthy habits.

ASIAN DIETS

Traditional Asian diets vary dramatically from the typical American diet. To begin, chopsticks are used instead of forks or knives. Using chopsticks often helps an individual eat more slowly. Smaller plates are often used as well, which also helps to curb portion size.

Many traditional Asian diets revolve around carbohydrates such as rice or pastas at each meal. Many of these carbohydrates, for example, white rice, are not whole grains. Asian diets regularly include fish and avoid red meat as their protein sources. Dairy products are not typically included in Asian diets.

With Asian diets, hot teas are often consumed before a meal, and consumption during meals of such cold beverages as water or calorie-dense sodas is avoided.

Asian diets tend to be low in saturated fat and emphasize nonstarchy vegetables at each meal. Asian plates often contain 2-3 times more vegetables than meat. Asian diets are high in fiber and use vegetables to contribute satiety and fullness. Dessert is saved for special occasions and used sparingly.

To adapt your Asian meals, choose 1 carbohydrate serving per meal and focus on whole grains. Substitute brown rice for white rice, or whole-wheat pasta for white pasta. This means no more than ½ cup brown rice or whole-wheat pasta per meal. Note that this should be your only carbohydrate for the meal. Incorporating fish contributes lean protein and healthy fats to meals.

For Thai food, coconut milk is often used as a curry base. To reduce the fat content of the meal, substitute light coconut milk. Avoid peanut sauce because of its high calorie content. Tofu is often used as a protein source, and if you select a low-fat or light tofu, it aligns well with the 20/20 LifeStyles plan. To reduce calories in curries or stir-fry dishes, limit oil to 1 teaspoon in meal preparation.

Substitute low-sodium soy sauce, or avoid it completely if you have high blood pressure. Consuming more fish than red meats is an acceptable substitution. Focusing on 3 or more vegetable servings at meals will help contribute volume and overall satiety.

Here are some Asian-inspired recipes to try:

Thai Chicken Satay with Peanut Sauce

Sauce:

- ☐ 5 dried red chiles
- ☐ ¼ teaspoon ground coriander
- ☐ ¼ teaspoon ground cumin
- ☐ ½ teaspoon kosher or sea salt
- ☐ 1 garlic clove, minced
- ☐ 1 tablespoon minced peeled lemongrass
- ☐ 1 tablespoon minced peeled fresh ginger
- ☐ 1 tablespoon minced shallots or red onion
- ☐ ¾ cup light coconut milk
- ☐ 2 tablespoons creamy all-natural peanut butter
- ☐ 1 tablespoon brown sugar
- ☐ 2 tablespoons fresh lime juice
- ☐ 1 tablespoon fish sauce

Marinade:

- ☐ 1 cup light coconut milk
- ☐ 3 tablespoons minced shallots or red onion
- ☐ 2 tablespoons low-sodium soy sauce
- ☐ 1 tablespoon minced peeled fresh ginger
- ☐ 1 teaspoon ground turmeric
- ☐ 1½ pounds chicken breast, trimmed and cut diagonally into thin slices
- ☐ Cooking spray

Directions:

- To prepare sauce, place chiles in a small bowl and cover with hot water. Let stand 30 minutes.

- Drain and finely chop chiles.

- Combine coriander, cumin, salt, and garlic in small bowl and stir to form a paste. Add chiles, lemongrass, ginger, and shallots, one at a time, until each ingredient is incorporated into paste.

- Heat ¾ cup coconut milk in a small saucepan over medium heat. Add paste mixture and cook for 1 minute. Stir in the peanut butter until smooth. Add brown sugar, lime juice, and fish sauce; cook 1 minute. Remove from heat; cool.

- To prepare marinade, combine 1 cup coconut milk and the next 4 ingredients (shallots through turmeric) in a large plastic zip-top bag. Add chicken to bag. Seal and marinate in refrigerator 45 minutes.

- Remove chicken from bag; discard marinade. Thread chicken slices evenly onto 12 6 inch skewers.

- Prepare grill or sauté pan.

- Place skewers on grill rack or sauté pan coated with cooking spray and cook for 5 minutes on each side or until done. Serve with sauce.

Serves 4 (serving size: 3 skewers and ¼ cup sauce). Per serving: Calories 360, fat 11 g, protein 43 g, fiber 1 g.

Curried Tofu

Sauce:

- ☐ 1 cup light coconut milk
- ☐ 2 tablespoons chopped fresh cilantro
- ☐ 1 teaspoon red curry paste
- ☐ ½ teaspoon brown sugar
- ☐ ½ teaspoon salt

Tofu and Vegetables:

- ☐ Cooking spray
- ☐ 2 12 ounce packages extra-firm low-fat or light tofu
- ☐ 4 cups baby spinach
- ☐ 1 medium red bell pepper, sliced

Directions:

- To prepare sauce, whisk all 5 ingredients together in a small bowl.

- Drain, rinse, and pat dry tofu. Slice block crosswise into 8 inch slabs. Coarsely crumble each slice into bite-size pieces. Heat large nonstick skillet over medium-high heat, coat with cooking spray, and add tofu pieces in a single layer. Do not stir for 5 minutes or until tofu browns. Then gently stir and continue cooking, stirring occasionally, until all sides are golden brown. Add spinach, bell pepper, and curry sauce and cook until heated through, 1-2 minutes.

Serves 4 (serving size: 1½ cups). Per serving: Calories, 269, fat 14 g, protein 20 g, fiber 5 g.

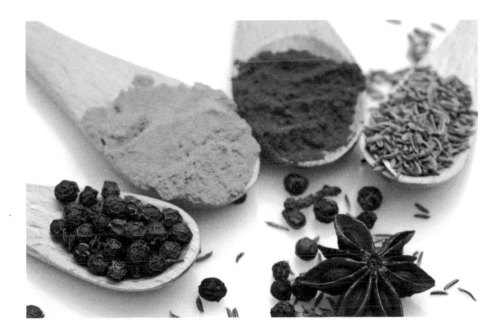

INDIAN DIETS

Many traditional Indian diets are vegetarian and contain large quantities of carbohydrates. Curries, a common Indian dish, include a sauce with vegetables and other items. Curry sauces can have a base of tomato, cream, or coconut milk or can be a thick, gravy-like concoction. Curries vary by region and come in many varieties. Some curries are made with protein and tofu as the main ingredients, others with a nonstarchy vegetable such as eggplant or a starchy vegetable such as potato. Curries are often served alongside breads, rice, or legumes.

Some regions of India include fish as a protein source; others include such higher-fat meats as lamb and beef. Meats can often be cooked in a type of clarified butter called ghee. Legumes and grains constitute a majority of Indian dishes. Dahl is a dish made from lentils, which along with chickpeas is a diet staple in many regions of India. Indian leavened breads, such as naan, roti, and chapatti are common meal staples as well. Indian diets can also feature fried or stuffed breads, for example, samosas, which are high in both fat and calories.

Dairy is used in the form of fermented yogurts such as raita and lassi. Paneer, similar to cottage cheese, is used to contribute protein to meals. Yogurt- and cream-based sauces are also common dairy-based foods in the Indian diet. Pickled fruits and vegetables, or chutneys, are used as sauces or atop protein. Chutneys are also made from fresh or dried fruits and spices.

Flavorful Indian dishes may use many non-salt based spices such as turmeric, ginger, garlic, chiles, or black pepper. Many dishes are cooked in oil or ghee. Reducing the oil used for cooking while keeping all the traditional flavorful spices can help make Indian dishes healthier.

To adapt your meals to the 20/20 LifeStyles plan, your meals must be centered on lean protein, for example, fish or low-fat tofu, and nonstarchy vegetables. Tomato-based curries are healthier than the other coconut or cream-based curries. Limiting carbohydrates is crucial and, contrary to common beliefs, lentils and dahl are not considered protein sources but carbohydrates. Rice, chapatti, and other Indian breads, along with fruit, are all carbohydrates as well. Select only ONE of these items to include at a meal, and limit quantities to 100 calories. This may only be ½ cup of dahl, or ½ of a roti or chapatti. Be mindful of portions with Indian breads. One slice or piece can be as much as 200-300 calories.

Making raita with Greek yogurt will help increase protein, and paneer can be made with nonfat or low-fat milk. Such non-curry dishes as tandoori chicken, tikka masala, or meat-based skewers are choices that align well with your healthy meal plan. Select chicken or seafood for lower-calorie protein options than beef or lamb. Avoid dishes made with ghee and heavy cream-based sauces, and if chutneys are used, limit portions to 1 tablespoon.

Here are some lighter versions of Indian dishes that fit the 20/20 LifeStyles plan.

STAGE 2

Indian-style Scrambled Eggs

Ingredients:

- ☐ 1 teaspoon olive oil
- ☐ ¼ medium onion, chopped
- ☐ 4 egg whites
- ☐ Pinch of turmeric
- ☐ Pinch of chili powder
- ☐ Pinch of ground cumin
- ☐ Pinch of garam masala
- ☐ Pinch of fresh ginger, chopped
- ☐ 1 medium tomato, chopped
- ☐ ½ cup leafy greens

Directions:

- Heat nonstick frying pan over medium-high heat and add olive oil.
- Add onions and allow them to turn light brown.
- Add ginger and tomatoes.
- In bowl, mix egg whites and seasonings and whisk.
- Reduce heat under pan to medium-low and pour in egg mixture.
- Stir eggs until they form soft curds.
- Add leafy greens to egg mixture and stir until wilted.

Serves 1. Calories 149, fat 5 g, carbohydrate 12 g, protein 17 g.

From TLC by Kelly Rossiter (October 2009), http://recipes.howstuffworks.com

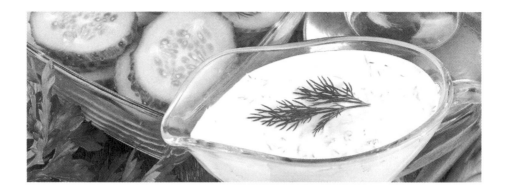

STAGE 3

Cucumber Raita

Ingredients:

- ☐ 2 cups plain fat-free Greek yogurt
- ☐ 1 cucumber, chopped
- ☐ 1 teaspoon roasted cumin powder
- ☐ Few sprigs of cilantro
- ☐ ½ cup vegetables (carrots, celery, cucumbers)
- ☐ Chili powder and ground pepper (optional)

Directions:

- Stir together yogurt and spices, mix until smooth.

- Add chopped cucumber and cilantro to mixture.

- Mix 1 serving of healthy fat (10 olives, or 1 tablespoon sunflower seeds, pumpkin seeds, or sesame seed, or 6 almonds) into cucumber raita.

- Use as dip for vegetables.

Serves 2. Per serving: Calories 137, fat 5 g, carbohydrate 9 g, protein 14 g.

From Chef in You by DK (April 2011), http://chefinyou.com

STAGE 5

Eggplant Curry With Yogurt

Ingredients:

- ☐ 3 eggplants, cubed
- ☐ 2 garlic cloves, minced
- ☐ 1 tablespoon ginger, grated
- ☐ 1 onion, diced
- ☐ ¼ teaspoon cardamom
- ☐ ¼ teaspoon cumin
- ☐ ¼ teaspoon mustard seed
- ☐ 1 teaspoon garam masala
- ☐ 1 teaspoon turmeric
- ☐ ⅓ cup Almond Breeze Unsweetened Coconut milk
- ☐ 1 6 ounce container plain fat free Greek yogurt
- ☐ ½ tablespoon canola or olive oil
- ☐ 1 scoop referred protein powder (not calculated in the nutritional facts)

Directions:

- Combine onion, garlic, and ginger in oil and add all spices.
- Stir in eggplant cubes. Add almond milk and cook for 10-15 minutes.
- Remove from heat.
- Mix protein powder with yogurt and stir into mixture.

Serves 4. Calories 125, fat 5 g, carbohydrate 15 g, protein 5 g

From Cooks United by Dialog (November 2008), http://www.cooksunited.co.uk

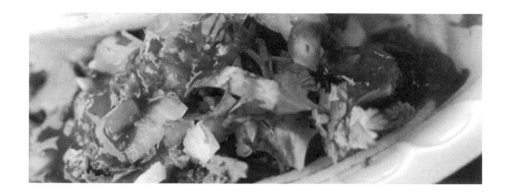

HISPANIC DIETS

The Hispanic diet features cuisines from many regions and is influenced by many cultures across the world. Diets vary dramatically by region, each country using different types of meal staples, proteins, and spices in varying quantities. Mealtimes vary in these cultures, but all of them put an emphasis on taking time to enjoy a meal. For example, in Spain, dinner may not be eaten till 9:00 p.m. or later, and since lunch is in the afternoon, many Spaniards will have tapas, or small appetizers and snacks between their lunch and dinner meals.

The mainstays of many Latin American dishes are corn, beans, chili peppers, and tomatoes. European influences led to the introduction of poultry, beef, and dairy products. Such spices as cumin and herbs such as cilantro are commonly used to flavor dishes. Chiles and peppers (jalapeno, habanero, pasilla, poblano) are flavorful components of the meals as well.

In many regions, fish and seafood are the primary source of protein. Spanish cuisine features rice or pasta and such seafood-based dishes as paella. More exotic proteins, for example, octopus and eel, are used as well. Spanish tapas include items such as spiced meats and olives, fish in olive oil, and seafood in tomato-based sauces.

Puerto Rican cuisine uses more starchy tropical tubers, such as taro and cassava, in cooking. Peppers are also common ingredients, along with numerous fresh herbs. Proteins used include sausages, salamis, duck, oxtail, and beef and chicken.

Traditional Mexican dishes feature corn as well as beans, avocado, vanilla, and cocoa. Grain and meats are often served together instead of separately, in such dishes as tacos, burritos, soups, and stews. Beans are a staple of many dishes. Grains such as maize and grain-based corn tortillas are ingredients in tacos, tamales, and arepas.

To adapt these diets to your plan, begin by centering your meal on protein and vegetables. Such items as fajitas can be great choices when dining out or cooking at home. Enchiladas, burritos, and tamales should be avoided because of their very high calorie content. Instead of flour tortillas, which are often made with lard, corn tortillas make the better choice. Limit such carbohydrates as beans or rice to 100 calories, or 1 serving per meal, and increase the quantity of vegetables in the dish. When cooking at home, make sparing use of such higher-fat Mexican cheeses as queso fresco or cotija.

Contemporary Hispanic diets have been impacted by the American diet. So-called Mexican food is in fact the Americanized Tex-Mex version, featuring enormous plates full of rice, beans, and cheese. This change has turned a balanced traditional meal into a calorie and carbohydrate laden disaster. If you must dine out at a Mexican restaurant, select fajitas, or another protein and vegetable based dish. To avoid unwanted calories, stay away from the rice, beans, and chips usually served.

Here are some Latin-inspired recipes with protein as the main ingredient. Stage 2 Option: Serve over lettuce and top with salsa OR Stage 3 Option: Serve over lettuce and top with salsa and fat-free sour cream.

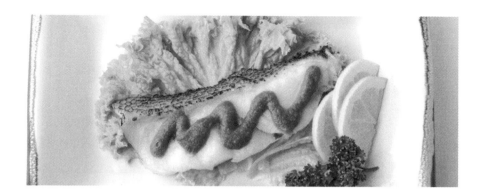

Spicy Cod

Ingredients:

- ☐ 1½ tablespoons low-fat mayo
- ☐ ½ teaspoon paprika
- ☐ ½ teaspoon garlic powder
- ☐ ½ teaspoon onion powder
- ☐ ¼ teaspoon pepper
- ☐ ⅛ teaspoon oregano
- ☐ ⅛ teaspoon ground thyme
- ☐ 1 tablespoon lemon juice
- ☐ 1 pound cod fillets

Directions:

- Preheat oven to 350° F.

- Thaw fish if frozen. Place fish fillets on a baking pan.

- Combine spices and mayo in small bowl. Spread evenly over fish.

- Bake until fish flakes, approximately 20-25 minutes.

Serves 3. Per serving: Calories 86, fat 1 g, carbohydrate 1 g, protein 17 g.

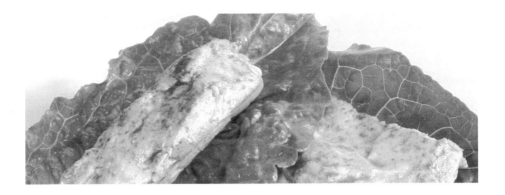

Spicy Chicken

Ingredients:

- ☐ 1⅓ pounds boneless, skinless chicken breasts
- ☐ 3 cups low-sodium chicken broth
- ☐ ¼ teaspoon Tabasco sauce
- ☐ ½ teaspoon chili powder
- ☐ 1 tablespoon red pepper flakes
- ☐ 1 teaspoon paprika
- ☐ 1 tablespoon seeded and minced jalapeno pepper (optional)

Directions:

- In a large stockpot, combine all ingredients and bring to a boil for 5 minutes. Reduce heat to low, cover, and simmer for 40 minutes. Uncover and simmer for 20 minutes.

- Remove pot from heat and set aside for 1 hour. Remove chicken and shred.

Serves 4. Per serving: Calories 180, fat 2.5 g, carbohydrate 2 g, protein 36 g.

APPENDIX L

HEALTHY DINING AT ETHNIC RESTAURANTS

Dining out healthfully can be challenging, because restaurant meals are often high in sodium and calories. To help you make healthy choices, we have listed some guidelines to follow and specific dishes to order when dining out. Remember, protein- and vegetable-centered dishes will always be the best options and the easiest meals to track. Always ask how an item is prepared; avoid heavy sauces, gravies, and dressings; and ask for all items to be prepared without butter or oil.

THAI

Good Choices:

Stir-fry entrées with chicken, seafood, tofu, and a variety of vegetables cooked with basil, Thai spices, lime juice, lemongrass, curry paste, or chili paste.

- Satays (meat skewers)

- Larb gai salad (chicken salad, served warm)

- Side of brown rice (½ cup = 100 calories)

Again, ask for your entrée to be prepared without extra butter or oil.

Avoid:

- Dishes with curry sauce (coconut milk)

- Panangs (these sauces are very calorie dense)

- Dishes made with peanut sauce

406

- Noodle dishes such as pad Thai.
- White rice

ITALIAN

Good Choices:

- Chicken piccata and cacciatore
- Steamed mussels and clams without butter sauce
- Salads with chicken, dressing on the side
- Cioppino (a broth-based fish stew)

Avoid:

- Pizza and pasta dishes, many of which (manicotti, ravioli) are full of cheese and therefore very high in carbohydrates and fat
- Dishes with cream sauces
- Breaded meats

MEXICAN

Good Choices:

- Fajitas (chicken, beef, shrimp) with vegetables
- Salad with lean meat, vegetables, salsa, and guacamole (limit 2 tablespoons)
- Carne asada with lettuce and salsa
- Soft corn tortillas, which are lower in calories than flour (2 corn tortillas = about 100 calories). Limit to 2 small tortillas

Avoid:

- Chips and salsa (ask the waiter to remove them from your table)

- Rice and bean side dishes (enchiladas, nachos, burritos, tamales are all high in calories) Deep-fried preparations, such as chimichanga

INDIAN

Good Choices:

- Tandoori chicken (without skin)

- Chicken or shrimp vindaloo

- Fish or lean meat kebabs

- Lentil dahl (limit ½ cup serving)

- Raita (cucumber yogurt sauce), small portion only

* Ask for dishes to be prepared without extra butter or oil.

Avoid:

- Dishes with coconut milk or cream base

- Curry dishes, which can be very calorie dense

- Breads

- White rice

- Fried items, such as samosas

JAPANESE

Good choices:

- Sashimi

- Nigiri

- Stir-fried entrées with chicken, seafood, tofu with vegetables

- Edamame (½ cup = 100 calories)

- Side of brown rice (½ cup = 100 calories)

  * *Use small amounts of soy sauce, and choose low-sodium soy sauce if it is an option.*

Avoid:

- All tempura and deep-fried items

- Sticky white rice

STEAK OR SEAFOOD RESTAURANTS

Good Choices:

- Broiled or grilled filet mignon, sirloin steak

- Fish prepared without butter or oil

- Extra vegetables or salad with dressing on the side

  * *Ask that the meat be grilled without butter or oil*

Avoid:

- Sauces and gravies

- High-calorie salad dressings

- High-calorie side dishes, such as mashed potatoes

APPENDIX M

ALTERNATIVE SNACK OPTIONS

These snack options are listed by the stage of the meal plan. Note that there is no listing for additional snack options for Stage 2 or Stage 7. Stage 2 snacks are the same as Stage 1, and Stage 7 allows grain-based foods only at meals, not for snacks. If you are on Stage 7, you can chose from any stage on this list.

Balanced snacks should contain:

- 150-250 calories

- 15-30 grams carbohydrate paired with

   › 2 ounces very lean protein and/or

   › 5-10 grams heart-healthy fat

The snack ideas below conform to these standards.

STAGE 1	CALORIES	FAT (g)
20/20 LifeStyles Protein Bar	220-240	8-10
2 ounces very lean protein plus 1 cup berries	130	0-2
20/20 LifeStyles Ready-To-Drink shake plus 1 cup berries	220	6
20/20 High Protein Dry Powder Shake plus 1 cup berries (*NO peanut butter*)	260	0

STAGE 3	CALORIES	FAT (g)
1 cup nonfat or low-fat plain Greek yogurt plus 1 cup berries	130-150	0-2
2 low-fat string cheeses plus 1 cup berries	180-200	5

STAGE 4	CALORIES	FAT (g)
½ cup nonfat or low-fat cottage cheese plus ½ cup fruit	160-180	0-2
1 cup nonfat or low-fat plain Greek yogurt plus ½ cup fruit	140-170	0-4
2 Light Laughing Cow cheeses plus ½ cup fruit	165	7

STAGE 5	CALORIES	FAT (g)
1 cup nonfat flavored Greek yogurt plus 1-2 tablespoons of nuts or seeds	140-220	5-10
½ cup nonfat or low-fat cottage cheese plus ½ cup nonfat or low-fat flavored yogurt	190-220	0-4
½ cup nonfat or low-fat flavored yogurt plus 1 low-fat string cheese	170-200	0-6

STAGE 6	CALORIES	FAT (g)
½ cup nonfat refried beans plus ¼ cup melted low-fat cheddar cheese	150-170	4-6
¼ cup hummus plus ½ cup mixed vegetables	130	4-6
Halved whites of 2 hardboiled eggs filled with 4 tablespoons hummus	135	4-6

APPENDIX N

VITAMINS AND SUPPLEMENTS

One of the most important nutritional supplements is fish oil. We call it the fountain of youth, because it can slow the aging process and prevent many metabolic disorders. It helps prevent heart disease, type 2 diabetes, and high blood pressure, as well as several other harmful conditions. The protective powers of fish oil were noted by a Danish scientist, who observed that the Greenland Eskimos had an exceptionally low incidence of heart disease and arthritis, despite a diet very high in fat-whale blubber.

Researchers found that fish is very high in two essential fatty acids-EPA and DHA. They're called essential fatty acids because, although our bodies cannot make them, they're essential in preventing aging of our cells and hardening of our arteries. These fatty acids are polyunsaturated and grouped into two families: omega-6 and omega-3. Omega-6 fatty acids actually harm the body by causing inflammation that can damage arteries, cause blood clotting (strokes), and increase tumor growth. Omega-3 fatty acids do just the opposite and are protective of your body. Although we need both of these fatty acids, it's vital to limit the intake of omega-6. We recommend two soft-gel 20/20 LifeStyles concentrated capsules daily. That amount will give you 600 mg of EPA and 400 mg of DHA, meeting the requirement to keep your omega-6 and omega-3 ratio close to a healthy ratio. If you buy your fish oil elsewhere, make sure it has adequate EPA and DHA. It's also important to make sure it's purified, fresh, and free of heavy metals that can come from bottom fish.

In addition, it's important to know that when you consume any fats, you create free radicals in your bloodstream, which can damage arteries. So we also recommend that you take antioxidant vitamins, such as vitamin E, along with the fish oil (36).

Vitamin D is probably the most important vitamin to discuss. Vitamin D appears to help with insulin secretion, blood pressure, and immune system function, as well as prevention of certain types of cancer. We've found that most of our 20/20 LifeStyles participants are low in this vitamin. Although our bodies produce vitamin D from sunlight, the sunscreen we use to prevent skin cancers also limits the amount of vitamin D we produce. If you live in a sunny climate and are outdoors a great deal of the time, you probably don't need to take additional vitamin D. For adults, we recommend 600 IU daily, and for seniors, 800 IU daily.

The Food and Drug Administration publishes a recommended daily value (DV) for all vitamins, listed on nutritional supplements and foods. We aren't satisfied with these values because they haven't been updated since 1970, even though later studies have since recommended different values many times.

Most of us have heard about folic-acid deficiencies related to birth defects. But folic acid does much more than prevent spina bifida in newborns. Homocysteine is an amino acid found in the blood, and high levels of homocysteine cause hardening of the arteries and dementia. Simply taking 300 mcg of folic acid daily can prevent high homocysteine levels in your body.

Vitamin C, a powerful antioxidant, has been found to lower the risk of cataract formation and hardening of the arteries. We recommend 200 mg of vitamin C daily.

There are water-soluble vitamins and fat-soluble vitamins. If you take too much of a water-soluble vitamin, it will just be eliminated in your urine. However, if you take too much of the fat-soluble vitamins,

36. See video Fish Oil-The Fountain of Youth under Lifestyle Series in Appendix J.

you may become toxic. Vitamin C is water soluble, so any excess will be eliminated from your body. Hence some people take very high doses with no harm to themselves. Vitamin E is fat soluble, however, so you should not take more than 200 IU per day.

Beta carotene, also fat soluble, is converted to vitamin A by our bodies. Taking vitamin A directly can cause toxicity, but that does not occur with beta carotene. Beta carotene helps with vision, aids the immune system, and promotes healthy skin, hair, bones, teeth, and nails. We recommend 2000 IU of beta carotene daily.

We have already mentioned one of the B vitamins, folic acid. Two others, B6 and B12, protect arteries, stop nerve damage, slow aging, and help protect us from cancer. We recommend 20 mg of B6 and 1200 mcg of B12 daily.

Coenzyme Q-10 improves muscle condition (including heart muscle), skin, and gums. We recommend 100 mg daily.

Alpha lipoic acid, also an antioxidant, is critical for energy production at the cellular level. It helps to activate the insulin receptors and therefore combats insulin resistance. We recommend 50 mg daily.

Minerals are also important to keep your body in balance and working properly. The average American only gets 60-80 percent of the required daily amount of calcium. If you exercise, you lose more calcium in your perspiration. We recommend 600 mg daily. Since calcium and iron are absorbed in the same pathway, they should not be taken at the same time of day.

Iron is necessary in the production of red blood cells, which carry oxygen to all your cells. Premenopausal women should take 10 mg per day. Men and postmenopausal women usually require no iron supplementation.

Zinc is another mineral most people have too little of. Zinc helps with fat burning, helps build protein and muscle, prevents certain eye problems, helps the immune system, and protects the nervous system. You lose zinc when you exercise and perspire. We recommend 11 mg daily.

Magnesium is necessary for heart function, effectiveness of the body's insulin, bones, and teeth. We recommend 200 mg daily.

These are the basics. You can find out more by viewing the following videos in Appendix J:

Fish Oil-"The Fountain of Youth"

Vitamins and Minerals 1

Vitamins and Minerals 2

If this all seems a bit complicated, you can purchase your vitamins and supplements in handy daily packets at:

https://shop.2020lifestyles.com/c-4-supplements.aspx

INDEX

ABOUT THE AUTHOR
Dr. Mark Dedomenico

Dr. Mark Dedomenico, a former cardiovascular surgeon, played a key role in developing the procedure known as Coronary Bypass Surgery along with Dr. Lester Sauvage. Working together as two of the initial founders of the Hope Heart Institute, they also created some of the most significant developments in heart surgery. These included the creation of artificial heart valves and Bionit arterial grafts used to replace damaged or atherosclerotic arteries. Dr. Dedomenico's work has also taken him into the areas of genetics, nutrition, exercise physiology, and behavior modification.

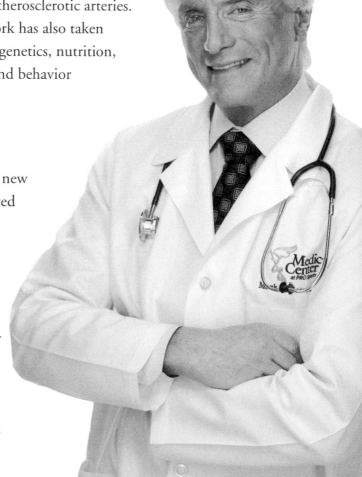

In 1992, Dr. Dedomenico began a new research project devoted to the treatment of early stage metabolic disease to prevent individuals from later needing cardiovascular surgery or medications to control hypertension, high cholesterol and diabetes. The research led to the creation of the 20/20 LifeStyles program. In 2002, 20/20 LifeStyles was selected as a credentialed provider of Microsoft's weight-management program.

Dr. Dedomenico's research and work with 20/20 LifeStyles remains ongoing and prevalent. He has formulated successful long term treatment methods of obesity, hyperlipidemia, hypertension, diabetes, depression, fibromyalgia, binge eating disorders and arthritis. Additionally, Dr. Dedomenico is currently involved in a major osteoarthritis research project in conjunction with Colorado State University. He is devising new methods to control, prevent and stop the disorder.

In addition to his experience as a practicing surgeon, Dr. Dedomenico spent many years overseeing one of the country's largest and most respected privately-held companies, Golden Grain Macaroni Company, the producer of many well-loved consumer products, including Rice-a-Roni, Mission and Golden Grain pasta, Ghirardelli chocolates, and Vernell candies.